Carnivore Diet for Women

Everything a woman needs to know about the carnivore diet.

Claudia Drake

Disclaimer

The information provided by Carnivore Diet for Women ("we," "us" or "our") is for general information only. All information is provided in good faith, however we make no representation or warranty of any kind, express or implied, regarding the accuracy, adequacy, validity, reliability, availability or completeness of any information. Under no circumstance shall we have any liability to you for any loss or damage of any kind incurred as a result of the use of any information provided. Your use of the site and your reliance on any information is solely at your own risk.

The book may contain links to other sites or content belonging to or originating from third parties or links to websites and features in banners or other advertising. Such external links are not investigated, monitored, or checked for accuracy, adequacy, validity, reliability, availability or completeness by us. We do not warrant, endorse, guarantee, or assume responsibility for the accuracy or reliability of any information offered by third-party websites linked through the book or any website or feature linked in any banner or other advertising. We will not be a party to or in any way be responsible for monitoring any transaction between you and third-party providers of products or services.

The book cannot and does not contain medical/health advice. The medical/health information is provided for general information and educational purposes only and is not a substitute for professional advice. Accordingly, before taking any actions based upon such information, we encourage you to consult with the appropriate professionals.

The table of contents is empty because you aren't using the paragraph styles set to appear in it.

Table of Contents

Forward

Why write a book about the carnivore diet just for women? Because women are different from men!   Women have different metabolisms, different issues. Some of us "diet" for weight loss first, and health second. We usually lose weight more slowly. We are the ones who feed our families and teach them how to eat. And, lastly, because I am a woman.

Is the carnivore diet different for women?   Yes and no.   The basics of the carnivore diet are the same for both women and men. But it has a different effect on women because we have a different system and different perspectives. We may need to supplement vitamins and minerals if we don't eat "nose to tail" in order to fully support our female metabolism or if we come into this way of eating with severe deficiencies.

We deal with estrogen, progesterone and testosterone, as well as periods, PMS, menopause, depression, anxiety, PCOS, infertility, insulin sensitivity, anxiety, bipolar disorder, obesity, auto-immune diseases, diabetes, rheumatoid arthritis and multiple sclerosis among other things. These are concerns that can be improved, and some cured, through the information in this book.

I began my journey on the keto diet, and after several months, moved on to the carnivore diet. There were two reasons I changed to the carnivore diet. One, I couldn't control my urges for food on the keto diet. I ate small amounts of food and craved more and ate more. And more.

Second, I used artificial sweeteners and duplicated the sugary drinks and foods I had been eating before keto. Almond flour breads and cookies, as well as fat bombs, became a major force that weren't healthy for me and kept me from losing weight in a timely manner.   I couldn't control myself. Discovering information about the plant toxin oxalate sealed the deal for me. I converted to the full carnivore diet and didn't look back.

Switching to the carnivore diet brought control into my life. There were no more cravings for sweets or fruits. I was satisfied with the high nutrient, high fat, high protein foods I ate. I began intermittent fasting, eating only two meals a day, fasting from after dinner to noon the next day. And I started to slowly get healthier and lose weight.

The carnivore diet is considered to be a way of eating that leads to healing of the mind and body. It is not looked upon as a weight loss diet, even though almost everyone loses weight. It can improve not only physical ailments, but also improve mood disorders. It has truly led to a new way of life for me.

What is the Carnivore Diet?

The carnivore diet is a healing diet. It consists of eating animal products only—meat, poultry, fish, seafood, eggs, butter and full-fat dairy. An extreme version of the diet is red meat, water and salt. Consuming these foods will bring your body into ketosis, where you switch from burning sugar (glucose) for energy, to burning fat. Although this is a healing diet first, it is also a ketogenic diet and you will lose weight if you are overweight.

The difference between what is called the keto diet and the carnivore diet is the carnivore diet excludes all plants—fruits, vegetables, grains, nuts and seeds. It differs also in that while it is also high fat, it contains a higher level of protein than the keto diet.

The nutrients found in eating animal products to the exclusion of plants, coupled with the ability of ketones to re-regulate your immune system, provide your body with a better energy source than is available through glucose. The carnivore diet provides the healing power that is not found in a conventional ketogenic diet.

This is also an elimination diet. By eating only animal products you give your body a rest and provide it with mega-nutrients. Stopping all plant food instantly removes nearly all the allergens and anti-nutrients that cause some people health problems and discomfort.

Anti-nutrients are components found in plants that reduce the body's ability to absorb essential nutrients. Plants contain toxins. One of those anti-nutrients is oxalate and it can cause a lot of damage to your body. The nutrients you get from animal products to the exclusion of plants are more bioavailable due to the elimination of anti-nutrients.

There is currently only observation and anecdotal evidence as to the success and safety of the carnivore diet. Because the scientific mechanism of ketosis is the same in both keto and carnivore diets, I have used scientific studies on the ketogenic diet to demonstrate the current knowledge and value of ketosis actuated in the carnivore diet.

What can you eat?

The basic recipe for the diet is to "eat meat, drink water." By meat, I mean any animal, be it beef, pig, sheep, wild game, chicken, turkey, duck, fish, or shellfish. It also includes animal products such as heavy whipping cream, hard cheese, butter and eggs.

Ruminant animals, those with hooves, are the most nutrient dense. It's important to eat nose-to-tail to obtain the necessary vitamins, Offal, or animal organs such as liver, are packed with nutrients. Liver is sometimes referred to as "nature's multiple vitamin" and should be consumed once a week if possible. Many carnivores do not eat nose-to-tail and feel they do fine nutritionally, but I recommend a multiple vitamin or supplements for those who don't.

Eat cuts of meat that are high fat for the most part like rib eye, sirloin, strip, chuck steaks; prime rib, brisket roasts, and 80/20% hamburger When eating leaner meats, add butter or cook the meat in lard or bacon fat. Yes, bacon is allowed, but watch out for sugar as one of the first ingredients on the label.

Many carnivores eat grass-fed animal products and swear by them. Others maintain the importance of just eating animal products, whether they come from the grocery store or are high end grass fed. They point out all ruminant animals are basically grass fed the majority of their lives, and the difference is what they eat the last couple of months.

It's important to drink water, but not to go overboard and drink so much you flush out all your nutrients. I recommend the standard eight glasses of water a day. Some people add Redmond Real Salt to their water for extra electrolytes.

Because there are a lot of coffee drinkers in the carnivore community, even though coffee is a plant, it is "allowed." Coffee is very low in oxalate, an anti-nutrient, and many choose not to give it up. We're talking black coffee or with heavy whipping cream for those who are not dairy sensitive.

Eat until you are satiated, or full, but not stuffed. You are eating to meet your energy needs. Women usually eat between 1 1/2 and 2 pounds of meat a day depending on your size, activity level, and the type of meat you're consuming. You may want to consume more when eating meats of less nutrient density like chicken, e.g., when compared to beef. Eat the dark meat of poultry for the fat content, or add fat if eating white pieces such as chicken breast.

Cook your meat any way you like it. However, when cooking liver, it's important to cook it lightly as high heat destroys the available vitamin C content.

You can eat two or three meals a day, or eat as many carnivores do and practice intermittent fasting after your initial thirty days or so into the diet. In intermittent fasting, you eat only during a short window of time, e.g., 6 to 8 hours, and fast the remaining time. I engage in intermittent fasting, eating from noon to 6 pm, and fast the remaining time. This is a great way to add in even more health benefits.

Ketones and Ketosis

When you begin a carnivore diet, you are probably burning glucose for energy unless you have already been on a keto diet. By eliminating all glucose from your diet, your body will switch to burning fat. Your liver will convert the fat into ketones. This process is called ketosis. Beta-hydroxybuterate (BHB) is the most prevalent ketone, making up 70-80% of ketones in the blood. It is also produced as an exogenous ketone, a supplement produced from ketones, and sold in the marketplace.

Ketones are released into the bloodstream, taken up by the brain and other organs, and shuttled into the mitochondria, the powerhouse of the cell. Mitochondria convert calories from food into energy (ATP). Fat metabolism using ketones gives you more ATP molecules than those derived from glucose. A ketogenic diet is believed to improve biogenesis, a process by which cells increase mitochondrial mass (Hason-Olive). This increases your energy even more!

Ketones are accomplished players. They cause less oxidative stress to our body, a process which speeds up aging. They help kill cancer cells because cancer cells use glucose for fuel. Ketogenic diets have been used to treat and prevent epileptic seizures since 1923. They improve mood, have antidepressant-like effects and may be beneficial in preventing neurodegenerative diseases. They lower inflammation and improve insulin sensitivity. And they increase fat loss while preserving muscle mass and performance.

Ketosis has shown benefits on a study on the role of ketogenic diets in Parkinson's and Alzheimer's diseases (Wlodarek), and cancer prevention (Klement, Weber). Exogenous ketones are also being considered in the treatment of psychiatric disorders (Kovacs). Studies also show the advantages for a ketogenic diet for multiple sclerosis (Brenton(a)), lupus (Youm), and Alzheimer's disease (Cunnane(c), Pinto, Broom).

Our brain connection to ketones has been evolutionary. Early humans developed with a significant layer of body fat on the fetus starting during the third trimester of pregnancy. By providing fatty acids for ketone production that are needed as brain fuel, this layer supports the brain's high energy needs well into childhood (Cunnane(d)).

While our brain uses glucose for fuel, its preferred fuel actually is ketones. Studies in humans show that brain glucose consumption decreases as ketone availability to the brain increases (Hasselbalch).

The role of ketones and ketosis in the carnivore diet goes far beyond eating meat and weight loss. It is pivotal to our overall, longterm health and well being, as well as constant new discoveries in the medical community.

Keto Flu and Electrolytes

At the beginning of the Carnivore Diet, there is a substantial shift in body water and electrolyte levels in the first few weeks. When you eliminate carbohydrates, that means your glycogen stores in your liver are depleted. Water is stored alongside glycogen, and as your glycogen stores are depleted, the body loses water.

As this water is expelled in urine, it takes out important minerals like calcium, potassium and magnesium that the body needs to function properly with it. This sets up an electrolyte imbalance. This imbalance can bring what is called the "keto flu" as you adapt to your new way of eating. Side effects can include muscle cramps, constipation, brain fog and low energy. Restoring the imbalance is imperative to avoid the keto flu, but also for optimal body functions.

Another source of the keto flu is carbohydrate withdrawal. You've been using carbs for energy previous to the carnivore diet. Switching to the carnivore diet puts you into ketosis where your body is burning fat for energy. Ketones are produced from all that fat burning.

Using carbs requires a different set of molecules and enzymes than ketone production. Before your body can switch over to ketones and use them as a source of energy, it has to first make more of some enzymes and less of others for a couple of days. This can make you feel tired and lethargic.

One way to make up for sodium loss is to salt your meals liberally, meaning, "salt to taste." The recommendation is 3-5 grams (3000-5000 mg) of sodium per day. One teaspoon is roughly 2 grams of sodium. Some people add Redmond Real Salt to their water for extra electrolytes.

General guidelines for potassium loss is anywhere from 1600 - 3000 mg per day (Cohn). The government Recommended Daily Allowance (RDA) for those on the standard American diet is 4700 mg! But it is likely carnivores need less potassium as it's believed they absorb their potassium at a higher rate. (See "Why Many Carnivores Don't Take Supplements, Appendix A.)

Potassium is often not at optimal levels in the general public, but if a woman on a carnivore diet is eating 1 1/2 to 2 pounds of pork or beef a day, in all probability she is getting a quantity of potassium that will meet her needs.

However, many people do choose to supplement for a variety of reasons. Many are not well when they begin a carnivore diet. It is recommended by some in the carnivore community that people supplement calcium, magnesium and potassium during the adaptation portion of the carnivore diet.

Sally K. Norton, a specialist in oxalates, suggests that those that may be experiencing "dumping" of oxalates when they quit eating plants also supplement. She recommends calcium citrate, potassium citrate and magnesium citrate.

I personally take a multiple vitamin because I do not eat organ meat (offal), as well as calcium citrate with D3, potassium citrate and magnesium citrate to deal with oxalates.

Anti-Nutrients

Anti-nutrients are compounds found in plant foods that essentially protect the plant. They are a plant's self defense mechanism. Their goal is to keep predators—humans and bugs—away. They do this by producing harmful chemical substances. They normally aren't immediately deadly, but often we have no idea the damage is being done to our bodies as we consume what we think is healthy.

These compounds are found in grains, legumes, beans, nuts, plant roots, vegetables, fruits, leaves, and seeds. They affect the absorption of nutrients from other foods eaten at the same time.

Some of the chemicals include lectins, which interfere with cellular functioning and are responsible for what's known as leaky gut. Saponins can also interfere with nutrient absorption and cause leaky gut and immune responses. Another is phytate which makes it impossible to soak up important minerals. Trypsin inhibitors impede the processes of digestive enzymes, and tannins interfere with iron absorption. Gluten causes gut distress and is difficult to digest. Glucosinolates are found in cruciferous vegetables such as broccoli and brussels sprouts. They can interfere with the absorption of iodine, which can interfere with thyroid function.

The anti-nutrient, oxalate, is an anti-nutrient that has been highlighted in the carnivore community. Oxalates are corrosive compounds in nano- and micro-crystal form that occur naturally in plants. Foods can be low or high in oxalates.

Examples of foods high in oxalate are beans, grains, bran, sesame and other seeds, peanuts, almonds, and other nuts, swiss chard, spinach, beets, potatoes, chocolate, rhubarb, figs, kiwi, blackberries, black pepper, cumin, and turmeric.

Examples of foods low in oxalate are meats, dairy, eggs, fats and oils, and other non-plant foods, arugula, avocado, bok choy, cabbage, cauliflower, cilantro, cucumber, garlic, kohlrabi, lettuce, mustard greens, mushrooms, green peas, and watercress.

This list is important because if you have been eating a high oxalate diet when you begin a carnivore diet, you will want to taper off of oxalates slowly.

Sally K. Norton, MPH, (www.SallyKNorton.com) advises oxalates cause both nutrient deficiencies and toxicity. They have been noted to cause weakened bones, connective tissues and fibrosis among other things. She believes there could be a connection to fibromyalgia and a host of other ailments.

Oxalates prevent nutrient absorption of iron, calcium and magnesium. They are enzyme inhibitors that can prevent proper digestion and cause gut and protein deficiencies. Oxalates collect in the body and irritate tissues. Almost all adults have some oxalate buildup in their body. A study of 182 normal thyroids found that 85% of people over age 50 have calcium oxalate crystals in their thyroid (Katoh).

Oxalates build up in your system and you may experience oxalate poisoning. When you stop consuming them you may experience oxalate "dumping" unless you taper off over a period of time. Everyone reacts differently, and you may have no reaction at all.

One of the many advantages of the carnivore diet is that it contains no anti-nutrients.

More complete information on oxalates can be found online at Facebook and Yahoo groups run by Susan Owens called Trying Low Oxalates and also at Sally K Norton's website (www.SallyKNorton.com).

An extensive eye-opening list of research studies on oxalates can be found in Appendix B.

Fats and Cholesterol

For years, fat was a four-letter word we were urged to ban from our diets. But fat is essential to human life and health. Fat is a major source of energy; it's stored energy. We can store months' worth of energy as fat, sometimes to our detriment!   And approximately 60% of our brain is made out of fat!

Fat helps absorb minerals and vitamins.   It's needed for building cell membranes and the sheaths surrounding nerves. It's essential for blood clotting, muscle movement and inflammation. It cushions our organs; it's a crucial component of our skin protecting us from the outside world.

Fats are important ingredients in tears, joint fluids and other slippery membranes. Certain essential vitamins, such as A, D, E, and K, all require fat in order to be absorbed by our intestines. There are a few fats, essential fatty acids, we absolutely must eat because we can't make them ourselves.

The more hydrogen atoms carried, the more "saturated" a fat is.   Saturated fat has more energy and has more calories per pound.   We have been led to believe saturated fats cause heart disease because of a 1970 study called "The Seven Countries Study," by a renowned scientist, Ancel Keys.

The study proved no causal link, and there have been numerous studies since showing no connection between saturated fat and heart disease (Chowdhury, de Souza, Siri-Tarino). There is much more evidence linking cholesterol disregulation and heart disease to refined carbohydrates than to saturated fats (Halton, Howard, Mente, Astrup, Jacobson).

Additional research shows that dietary cholesterol via eating a meat based diet promotes the repair of demyelinated lesions in the brain, like those found in MS patients. They also discovered "high" cholesterol is not associated with an increased risk of dementia (Mielke (a)).

Numerous studies found a possible relationship between low cholesterol levels and mood disorders, suicide ideation, and suicide attempts. Recent findings show that lowering plasma cholesterol by a plant based diet and statins *increase* depressive symptoms. Another study found women on lipid-lowering medication may be predisposed to aggression (Olson).

In "Eat Fat 2 Lose Fat," at (https://www.youtube.com/watch?v=BYCnpoa1Sdl), Dr. Ken Berry explains eating fat to lose fat. You want to lose the fat stored on your body, including the fat you carry inside of your heart, liver and your pancreas. The fat you carry inside your belly is much more dangerous to you than the fat you see in the mirror (Assuncao, Spadaro). Eating fat to lose fat actually works, (Sherman) and it's very healthy. On a ketogenic diet, you dial down the carbohydrates. On a carnivore diet, you dial the carbs to near zero.

Most of your sex hormones and your adrenal hormones come directly from cholesterol. You want lots of good saturated fat. Eating fat lowers your insulin level in your blood stream to low normal. Insulin helps your body store fat. Anytime your insulin is elevated, it's very hard to burn the fat you've already stored on your body. Anytime you eat carbohydrates, those carbs break down immediately into sugars. When the sugars hit your blood stream, your insulin goes up and that turns off your ability to meaningfully burn fat that you've already stored in or on your body. By eating little to no carbs on the carnivore diet and eating more healthy fats. you'll keep the insulin level at low normal.

Eating lots of healthy fats is going to raise your human growth hormone (HGH) level and your testosterone level in a good way. This is not going to make women masculine, it is going to move your HGH and testosterone into the optimal ranges so it makes it easier for you to burn the stored fat.

When you eat lots of healthy fat, you're going to make your brain work better You're going to be in a better mood, you won't be as anxious. You'll have more stamina and stability.

Although the body can build some saturated fat, it's better to eat good quality natural saturated fats in your diet. Saturated fats are found in red meat, whole-milk dairy foods and cheese. We thought for decades that total cholesterol was a marker of an increased risk of heart attack and stroke. That's why so many doctors told their patients to stop eating saturated fat or they would experience a heart attack. Or if you insisted on eating saturated fat, you had to take medicine that would lower your cholesterol.

Cholesterol does a lot of good things. It not only helps to prevent dementia, but protects against infectious disease. It has no bearing on heart disease, and even reduces the chance of death from all causes (Kaysen, Liang, Ravnscov (a)). Additionally, high cholesterol reduces Parkinson's risk (Anderson), the risk of dementia (Mielke (b)), lowers the risk of breast cancer (Paddock), and protects from infections and heart disease (Ravnscov (b)).

The carnivore diet plays an important part in your health for its role in the reduction of risk of diseases, protection, and brain and heart health. Only animal sourced foods provide cholesterol. It's not the fats and cholesterol that make a negative impact on one's lipid profile and risk factors, it is carbohydrates and sugars.

Fiber

It will probably surprise you to learn that fiber isn't necessary for nutrient and digestive health. And it turns out that low fiber intake is not associated with constipation. In a study of 63 people with constipation, eliminating fiber completely reversed their symptoms (Ho). People who decrease fiber decrease constipation. Another study noted a reduction in diverticula seen on colonoscopies on people who followed a low fiber diet (Peery). While fiber does decrease blood glucose, those on a carnivore diet avoid this issue by not eating sugar or items that reduce to glucose.

Another issue with fiber is that it is touted to potentially decrease cholesterol, and there's been a small effect noted with that. But we are discovering that cholesterol readings can change on a daily basis, and some believe they are meaningless. Others believe cholesterol is a measure of repair being facilitated in your blood vessels, and not a sign of distress.

A study showed a strong case *cannot* be made for a protective effect of dietary fiber against colorectal polyps or cancer (Tan). Nutritional psychiatrist, Dr. Georgia Ede asks the question, "Then why has fiber been so highly touted?" Dr. Ede believes scientists have assumed the difference in our traditional cultures and that of our modern cultures is lack of fiber rather than the addition of refined carbohydrates. "Fiber is not essential for human life or health," Ede states. "It doesn't get to the root of the problem." (htttps://www.diagnosisdiet.com/food/fiber/)

Depending on what kind of diet you have been on previously, when you start the carnivore diet, you will probably experience a change in bowel habits. A carnivore diet is a drastic reduction in fiber intake. You may experience a reduction or cessation in bowel movements for the first several days, especially if you've been consuming a lot of plant food previously. And you may not experience a bowel movement every day. If you're feeling fatigued and have gone for several days without a bowel movement, you may want to consider whether you are eating enough food. You might also benefit from fattier meats.

It is more likely you will experience loose stools or diarrhea in the early days of the carnivore diet. This is due to a higher intake of fat and no fiber to slow things down. This will calm down after a couple of days.

Vitamins

How do you get vitamins if you're not eating fruits and vegetables? Meat and animal products contain many of the necessary nutrients in a highly bioavailable form. The best way to optimize your diet is to eat abundant amounts of meat and animal products, and in doing so you will be removing oxalates and other anti-nutrients from your diet that block vitamin and mineral absorption.

According to the Department of Agriculture, beef contains potassium, vitamin D, iron, B-6, B-12, magnesium, selenium, zinc, niacin, phosphorus, choline, iron, and riboflavin. Liver is the queen of nutrients with potassium, vitamin A, B-6, magnesium, vitamin C, iron and B-12. Beef contains all nine essential amino vitamins.

Pork contains vitamins A, C, E, thiamin, riboflavin, niacin, B-6, folate, B-12, pantothenic acid, calcium, iron, magnesium, phosphorus, potassium, zinc, and copper.

Chicken contains niacin, selenium, B-6, phosphorus, choline, vitamin A, pantothenic acid, B-12, sodium, and folate.

Fish contains omega-3 fatty acids, vitamins A and D, riboflavin, calcium, phosphorus, iron, zinc, iodine, magnesium, and potassium.

What do these vitamins do for us? Iron in meat supports the nervous system; selenium helps protect cells from damage; Vitamins B-12 and B-6 help maintain brain function; zinc helps with a healthy immune system; phosphorus builds bones and teeth;

niacin supports energy production and metabolism; and riboflavin converts food into fuel.

Does the carnivore diet provide enough vitamin C for those on the diet? Given the RDAs have been set up for a general U.S. population consuming anti-nutrient rich plants which impede absorption of vitamins and minerals, the amount needed by those eating a carnivore diet may be much less.

Scurvy is the disease that results from a lack of Vitamin C. Symptoms of irritability and fatigue present after 8 to 12 weeks of inadequate intake of vitamin C. Symptoms include swollen, bleeding gums, loss of teeth, bruising, and rash.

There is a theory that because meat contains lots of glutathione, carnivores need less vitamin C (Rakowski). The fact is if people eating the carnivore diet were deficient in vitamin C, it would be apparent. However, clearly, there are no cases of scurvy in the carnivore community.

But we have to eat nose-to-tail in order to get the available vitamins. Not all of us eat offal, or organ meat, or consume quantities of seafood or dairy. We may or may not be consuming sufficient levels of biotin, folate, calcium, magnesium and vitamins A, C, and D, especially for those eating only beef. Some choose to supplement in this area.

Because I do not eat nose-to-tail, I choose to supplement my diet with a multiple vitamin. And because I believe I have a buildup of oxalates in my body contributing to fibromyalgia and possibly other ailments, I take magnesium citrate, potassium citrate and calcium citrate.

Our metabolism changes due to the effects of burning ketones for energy and eliminating plants from our diet. There are many healing attributes in the ketogenic diet, and it may be that the high nutrient values in the carnivore diet reduce the need for the RDA amounts of vitamins and minerals listed by the U.S. government. Many in the carnivore community believe so.

A carnivore viewpoint of vitamins, "Why Many Carnivores Don't Use Supplements," coupled with my comments, is included in Appendix A. Anecdotally, we are looking good, but there has been no scientific research to back up our views. It's up to each individual to choose for themselves as to whether or not to take a supplemental vitamin in accordance with their own health issues.

Intermittent Fasting

Intermittent fasting is a pattern of eating, a way of scheduling your meals. You are either digesting and absorbing food, or when you are not eating, you are fasting. It takes 12 hours of not eating to enter a fasted state. In a fasted state you are burning fat.

There are many ways of scheduling intermittent fasting. Probably the most popular is daily intermittent fasting. Pick out a six- or eight-hour period of time to eat, and fast the remaining period. I eat from noon to 6:00 pm and fast until noon the next day.

There is also weekly intermittent fasting where you can fast for one or more 24 hour periods. Alternate day intermittent fasting incorporates periods on alternate days.

Fasting has been described as a missing link in enhancing women's health. It can have powerful effects on your body and brain and may help you live longer (Barnosky, Longo). A 2016 overview on fasting showed it improved reproductive and mental health and slowed or prevented cancer and musculoskeletal disorders which are common in middle age and elderly women (Nair). The study found the role of fasting intervened in slowing or preventing metabolic dysfunctions common in elderly women.

Your cells initiate a cellular repair process with intermittent fasting. This includes autophagy where cells remove old dysfunctional proteins that build up inside cells. (Alirezaei, Kim).

By eating fewer meals, this leads to less caloric intake and intermittent fasting changes hormone levels to facilitate weight loss. In addition to lowering insulin and increasing growth hormone levels, it increases the release of the fat burning hormone norepinephrine (noradrenaline).

Intermittent fasting brings a plethora of benefits to couple with those of the ketogenic carnivore diet. Because of the metabolic changes in hormones, short term fasting may help increase your metabolic rate by up to 14% (Mansell, Zauner). Intermittent fasting helps you lose weight, eat fewer and burn more calories.

Other benefits of intermittent fasting include a decrease in inflammation (Johnson (a), Aksunger, Faris), and an increase in heart health (Varady, de Azevedo). Animal studies suggest intermittent fasting may prevent cancer (Descamps, Rocha). Intermittent fasting increases brain health and may aid in the growth of new nerve cells. It may also protect against Alzheimer's disease (Lee,J, Mattson). And intermittent fasting has been shown to extend life in rats (Carlson, Goodrick, Sogawa).

Exercise

What about exercise? Remember this is a way of eating, not a weight loss diet.   However, exercise is part of a good health program for any person whether they are on a diet or not. Proponents of exercise for the carnivore diet are split. Some say exercise is not necessary, especially at first, but to add light exercise such as walking later.   Others advocate a honeymoon period while one is getting adjusted to the diet, then add some level of walking or resistance training.

Still others believe exercise to not be necessary because it takes a toll on a body that needs to heal and that exercise can actually interfere with weight loss. So it depends on the individual, the state of your health, and your desire for activity. I advocate walking after adjustment to the diet.   Early exercise can be challenging if a person encounters the keto flu and you may experience initial weakness and tiredness while your body adjusts to this way of eating.

When and if you desire additional activity, light exercise or resistance training are great additions. Competitive or strenuous exercise usually requires the addition of carbohydrates and is incompatible with a strict carnivore diet, but may be part of an overall strategy.

Women and Hormones

The carnivore diet produces ketosis. Ketosis affects your hormones in a variety of ways. The hormones insulin, cortisol and thyroid, as well as the sex hormones, estrogen, progesterone, and testosterone are affected.

The following sections explain how ketosis found in the carnivore diet affects women's hormones and health in general.

Insulin

Insulin is a hormone made by your body's pancreas. It helps control the amount of sugar (glucose) in the blood. Insulin resistance and low insulin sensitivity are two similar issues that interfere with proper metabolism of glucose.

Insulin Resistance and Insulin Sensitivity

With insulin resistance, the body's cells don't respond normally to insulin. Glucose can't enter the cells as easily so it builds up in the blood.

Insulin sensitivity describes how sensitive a person is to the effects of insulin. It is a resistance to the hormone insulin, resulting in increasing blood sugar. We want to be insulin sensitive so that we require only small amounts of insulin to lower blood glucose levels.

When your insulin sensitivity is low, it puts increased pressure on your pancreas to increase insulin production to clear sugar from your blood.   Low insulin sensitivity may result in chronically high blood sugar levels.

Becoming insulin sensitive can bring about all sorts of metabolic wonders.   It decreases sugar cravings.   Your risk of cardiovascular disease, Alzheimer's disease and dementia is diminished; hot flashes or night sweats are reduced, and you rebuild bone health. You no longer have cravings and you look and feel healthy and energized.

Insulin resistance can have long term negative effects.   A 2015 study of young women with mild insulin resistance due to polycystic ovarian syndrome (PCOS) showed they had brain glucose uptake deficit resembling that of people in their 70s and 80s (Castellaro).   The mild insulin resistance was of interest because of its association with increased risk of Alzheimer's disease in middle aged and older adults (Ronnemaa , Craft, Matsuzaki, Schrijvers, Baker).

Results of the study of women with PCOS suggested that glucose disregulation and the development of a pattern of deteriorating brain glucose in older people can start in the second to third decade of life (Burns, Ishibashi).   Regional brain glucose hypometabolism (an abnormally low metabolic rate) can be present in those at risk of Alzheimer's disease due to old age, or to insulin resistance, regardless of age (Cunnane(a)).

Both insulin resistance and insulin sensitivity respond positively to a ketogenic diet, bringing blood sugar under control and contributing to a healthier life.

Polycystic Ovarian Syndrome (PCOS)

Women with polycystic ovarian syndrome (PCOS) have a hormone imbalance of too much luteinizing hormone (LH) and too little follicle-stimulating hormone (FSH). Over 50% are overweight or obese. Almost 70% of women with PCOS have an increased risk of insulin resistance and glucose intolerance.

Symptoms of PCOS include irregular menstrual cycles, infertility, weight gain, multiple cysts on ovaries, as well as excess facial and body hair. In addition, there may be signs of anxiety, panic attacks, mood swings, depression, fatigue and low sex drive due to the hormonal imbalance.

A ketogenic diet helps with weight loss and combating insulin resistance. As mentioned in the Insulin section, insulin resistance can be a serious situation leading to Alzheimer's disease. Lower body weight and decreased insulin resistance may be enough to balance your hormones, silence the PCOS and even get pregnant. A ketogenic diet has been known to decrease depression and improve anxiety, mood swings, and fatigue.

A 2005 study of women on a ketogenic diet suffering from PCOS showed there was significant weight loss and decreases in free testosterone, LH/FSH ratio and fasting insulin. Two women in the study became pregnant during the study despite previous infertility problems (Mavropoulos). A small study of four women resulted in weight loss and resumption of regular periods. Two of the women were able to conceive spontaneously (Alwahab).

Metabolic Syndrome

Metabolic Syndrome is a cluster of symptoms that appear together, increasing your risk of heart disease, stroke and type 2 diabetes. These conditions include increased blood pressure, high blood sugar, excess body fat around the waist and abnormal cholesterol or triglyceride levels.

Having just one of these conditions doesn't mean you have metabolic syndrome. But it does mean you may have a greater risk of serious disease. And if you develop more conditions, your risk of complications, such as type 2 diabetes and heart disease, rises even higher.

Metabolic syndrome is increasingly common, and up to 20-30% of middle aged women have it. It has been linked to the development of cardiovascular disease and diabetes (Bonora, Isomaa, Malik). Most of the disorders associated with metabolic syndrome don't have obvious signs or symptoms. Women tend to develop the disease ten years later than men, with a marked increase through the menopausal years (Janssen).

Intermittent fasting has evolved as a potential tool in redressing metabolic abnormalities as reported in various experimental studies (Ansom). Four weeks of intermittent fasting has been shown to reduce total weight, body mass index and waist circumference (Sadiya). A reduced waist circumference usually correlates with improved insulin sensitivity (Richelson). This signifies the role of fasting as an intervention in slowing as well as preventing metabolic dysfunction, which is common in elderly women.

Metabolic syndrome is closely linked to insulin resistance, as well as overweight or obesity and inactivity. Both the carnivore diet and intermittent fasting are beneficial for metabolic syndrome.

Obesity

More than two in three women in the United States are overweight or obese.   Women develop obesity when their body stores more calories than it uses over time.   Your body needs calories and essential vitamins, minerals and other nutrients to work properly.   But if your body stores more calories than it uses, your body will gain weight.

Being overweight or obese raises your risk for many serious health problems. Those include breathing problems, many types of cancers, diabetes, heart disease, high blood pressure, high cholesterol, pregnancy problems and stroke.

The safety and tolerability of a very low calorie ketogenic diet (less than 50 carbs/day) are a concern to some in the treatment of obese type 2 diabetes patients (Goday). This 2017 study evaluated the short-term safety and tolerability of a very low calorie diet. The conclusion was the interventional weight loss program based on a very low calorie diet was more effective in reducing body weight and improving glycemic control than a standard hypo, or low, caloric diet, with safety and good tolerance for type 2 diabetes patients.

Safety and success were also found in the long term effects of a ketogenic diet in obese patients. A study showed the ketogenic diet significantly reduced the body weight and mass index of the patients.   Further, it decreased the level of triglycerides, LDL cholesterol, and blood glucose, and increased the level of HDL cholesterol. Administering a ketogenic diet for a relatively longer period of time did not produce any significant side effects in the patients (Dashti).

Another study on the ketogenic diet relative to obesity in 2019 showed the effectiveness of the diet on weight loss, physical performance, cognitive function, eating behaviors and metabolic profile (Mohorko).

The carnivore diet, a ketogenic, low carb diet, although a healing diet first, will provide weight loss for those who need to lose weight.

Thyroid

Your thyroid produces thyroid hormones which control many activities in your body, including how fast you burn calories and how fast your heart beats. Diseases of the thyroid cause it to malfunction, making too much or too little thyroid. Women are more likely than men to have thyroid disease, especially right after pregnancy and after menopause.

Thyroid diseases can cause problems with your menstrual periods. Your thyroid helps control your menstrual cycle. Too much or too little thyroid will make your periods vary in intensity and regularity. Thyroid disease can also make your periods stop for several months or longer. If your body's immune system causes your thyroid disease, other glands, including your ovaries, may be involved. This can lead to early menopause—before the age of 40.

When thyroid disease affects your menstrual cycles, it also affects ovulation. You may have difficulty getting pregnant. Thyroid problems during the pregnancy can cause problems for both the mother and the baby.

Hypothyroidism is when your thyroid doesn't make enough thyroid. It slows down many of your body's functions. The most common cause of hypothyroidism in the United States is Hashimoto's disease. In this disease, the immune system mistakenly attacks the thyroid. This attack damages the thyroid so it doesn't make enough hormone.

Hyperthyroidism, or overactive thyroid, causes your thyroid to make more thyroid than your body needs. This speeds up your body's functions. The most common cause of hyperthyroidism is Graves' disease. It is also a problem with the immune system. Treatment with thyroid medication is usually a simple, safe and effective solution for thyroid disease.

The thyroid hormones function in almost every cell in the body. And diet can influence thyroid hormone levels and induce changes. A ketogenic diet can decrease circulating T3 hormone (Pasquali, Mathieson, Fontana), which can cause concern for some. But as Dr. Anthony Gustin (www.dranthonygustin.com/no-ketosis-does-not-ruin-womens-hormones) observes, a lowered T3 alone isn't the same thing as hypothyroidism.

Hypothyroidism is usually diagnosed with high levels of TSH and low levels of free T4. T3 is not part of the conversion process' of TSH and T4. When only T3 is decreased, your thyroid is "normal." In fact, a study has shown that lower levels of T3 show a benefit for preserving muscle mass and improving longevity (Baronawska).

Research shows a ketogenic diet can have an isolating effect on T3, and no effect on TSH or T4, so you're not hypothyroid with a lowered T3. (Fontana).

Cortisol

Cortisol can help control blood sugar levels, regulate metabolism, help reduce inflammation and assist with memory formulation. It has a controlling effect on salt and water balance and helps control blood pressure.

Cortisol is called the stress hormone in the body due to its role in stress response and other functions like breaking down fat and protein to make glucose. It's possible to have chronically high levels of cortisol if you don't control your stress levels, which are detrimental to your health and may lead to heart disease. One study found that cortisol increased over time in subjects given a ketogenic diet with a low/inadequate sodium intake (DeHaven), so it is important to keep your salt intake up.

Starting a ketogenic diet and removing carbohydrates from your diet forces your body to deal with carbohydrate withdrawal which is stressful. Your body has forgotten how to use fat as fuel and this can bring about the keto flu.

Ketones are a source of energy your body will love once adapted, and it's another option for your brain to use as fuel. It usually takes three to four weeks for your body to adapt, sometimes a little more. Once you become fat adapted, multiple studies show the levels of stress hormones are not higher than baseline (Volek(a), Volek(b)).

You can experience menstrual irregularities connected to increased cortisol. But once ketone adapted, your cortisol levels should drop (Miller), and your periods should become regular. If that doesn't happen, it could be due to outside stressors.

Estrogen, Progesterone and Testosterone

The ovaries produce estrogen, progesterone, and testosterone. Relatively small amounts of testosterone are released into your bloodstream by your ovaries and adrenal glands. Estrogen is also produced by the body's fat tissue. These sex hormones are involved in the growth, maintenance, and repair of reproductive tissues. They also influence other body tissues and bone mass.

Sex hormone release varies between night and day and from one stage of the menstrual cycle to another. Estrogen includes estriol, estradiol and estrone.

If your body produces too much testosterone, you may have irregular or absent menstrual periods. High levels can lead to infertility and are commonly seen in polycystic ovarian syndrome (PCOS). PCOS is an endocrine condition that is sometimes seen in women who have trouble getting pregnant. However, a systematic review has shown that low-carb (ketogenic) diets increase fertility in overweight and obese women (McGrice). Low carb diets also improve menstrual regularity and even pregnancy rates. PCOS is covered in more detail in a previous section.

Having too much fat on your body increases your estrogen levels. Fat tissue also functions as an endocrine organ, producing estrogen in fat cells. The more fat you have, the more estrogen your body makes. Estrogen overload can exacerbate hypothyroid issues, slowing metabolism and causing weight gain. If the estrogen overload comes from obesity in the first place, this becomes a vicious cycle of being overweight because you have thyroid problems and having thyroid problems because you're overweight.

Our bodies believe we need to stock up on fat for perceived future pregnancies. It wants to store fat at every opportunity.

Fortunately the evolution of birth control has changed the reality of continual pregnancies.

One of the advantages of the carnivore diet is the high level of protein. The results of a study of a high protein diet showed respondents had impressive hormone improvements, specifically a decrease in male hormones, a decrease in inflammation, and an improvement in insulin sensitivity (Mehrabani). Eating a high protein diet appears to contribute to hormonal healing.

Low fat intake because you're afraid of gaining weight can negatively impact your cycles. The dichotomy is that we have to remember to eat enough fat on the carnivore diet because we need it for enough nutrition and fat is energy! And good fats support hormone production and maintain hormone balance because they are the building blocks for estrogen, progesterone and testosterone. So, don't be afraid to eat fat!

Quick weight loss can cause a sharp drop in estrogen (Falsatti) which can cause missed periods. If you've had irregular periods, the carnivore diet can help to normalize them. At first you may get a heavier than normal flow, lasting longer than normal. Once your body adjusts to the changes in estrogen and fat storage, you can expect your period to return to normal.

Premenstrual symptoms, (PMS) can include everything from mood swings, brain fog, acne, backache, depression, fatigue, food cravings, and irritability. The carnivore diet often relieves many of the symptoms. Having too much estrogen can worsen PMS symptoms (Seippel). Often the underlying cause of PMS is estrogen dominance caused by having too much estrogen and not enough progesterone. Another cause of estrogen dominance is a diet high in sugar and refined carbohydrates.

Estrogen falls at menopause as a natural transition. On average menopause begins at 51 years of age. When it does, a woman produces less estrogen, progesterone, and testosterone. Lower levels of estrogen may increase a woman's risk for heart disease, stroke, osteoporosis and fractures.

Sex hormones, especially estrogens, possess antioxidant properties and play important roles in maintaining normal reproductive and non-reproductive functions. They exert brain protective actions and their loss during aging and natural or surgical menopause is associated with mitochondrial dysfunction, brain inflammation, synaptic decline, cognitive impairment and increased risk of age related disorders. (Zarate). Moreover, loss of sex hormones has been suggested to lead to signs of Alzheimer's disease.

Compensating for deteriorating brain energy metabolism is a core feature of an emerging strategy aimed at delaying the onset and/or progression of Alzheimer's disease. The brain's alternative source to glucose is ketones. Brain uptake of ketones appears to be normal in Alzheimer's disease (Cunnane (b)). It is thought ketogenic interventions in the form of a ketogenic diet or exogenous ketones (supplements) may delay Alzheimer's disease.

Studies show brain glucose consumption decreases as ketone availability to the brain increases (Hasselbalch). These results suggest that ketones are the preferred energy substrate for the brain because they enter the brain irrespective of glucose availability; if the energy needs of the brain are being increasingly met by ketones, glucose uptake decreases accordingly. This decrease in brain glucose uptake when both ketones and glucose are available supports the notion that ketones are the brain's preferred fuel.

Studies have shown attempting to treat the cognitive deficit early in Alzheimer's disease using ketogenic interventions such as MCT (medium chain triglycerides) supplements in clinical trials is safe, ethical and scientifically well-founded (Henderson, Rebello).

Menopause

Lucky us! We get hit with belly fat, brain fog, insomnia, memory loss, headaches, low libido, mood swings, and hot flashes. Estrogen, progesterone and testosterone all decline and ghrelin, the hunger hormone increases.

When we lose the protection of estrogen, our gut biome goes through a major shift. This also causes a reduction in neurotransmitter production, ultimately leading to chronic inflammation, a slower metabolism and poor sleep.

Ketones produced from a ketogenic diet such as the carnivore diet give us some relief. They give us better mental clarity and are believed to possibly work at preventing Alzheimer's disease. They can reverse insulin sensitivity, and there is less hunger due to the ghrelin effect. You have more energy because glucose highs and lows are stabilized. And you have more time because you can go for longer periods without eating. Nothing is greater than freeing up time from having to eat every couple of hours.

With menopause comes hot flashes. Although the origin of hot flashes are unknown, they are possibly related to low estrogen levels and their impact on the hypothalamus—a part of the brain that regulates temperature. Ketones created during ketosis help better feed and protect the brain and lower inflammation, which may in turn help regulate body temperature (Maalouf (a)).

And often libido goes right down the tube. Loss of libido may be a side effect of menopause due to fluctuating hormones. Sex hormones are made from fat. In fact, following a low-fat diet has been shown to *reduce* circulating estrogen (Rose) and could, in turn, actually reduce libido (www.perfectketo.com/menopause-diet/)). The opposite is true, eating a higher fat diet improves sexual function in women. The carnivore diet has been known to restore libido in women, even older women.

We gain weight when we hit menopause. That drop in estrogen contributes to the belly fat and obesity. We lose muscle mass, and we are burning less fat which brings about the weight gain. Also, many of us are on antidepressants, and they contribute to weight gain. But, once you get your hormones balanced, you will lose weight!

The high fat, ketogenic mechanisms of a carnivore diet can help you lose weight, control hot flashes, boost energy levels, fight insomnia and balance hormone levels to improve menopause symptoms.

Autoimmune Diseases

The health of your immune system dictates the health of every cell in your body. In the case of autoimmune diseases, your immune system starts to mistake healthy cells and tissues in your body as outside invaders. Examples are Hashimoto's thyroiditis, rheumatoid arthritis, lupus, Chrohns disease, multiple sclerosis and type 1 diabetes.

Your gut microbiome and the integrity of your gut lining both play a key role in whether or not you'll experience autoimmune disease (Kamada(a)(b)). An effective way to keep your gut happy is to reduce inflammation of the gut via the ketogenic diet. Ketone bodies in the form of beta-hydroxybutyrate (BHB) reduce overall inflammation, especially in your gut when you get into a ketogenic state (Youm).

The carnivore diet provides improvement in weight loss, heart health, inflammation and gut health for those who suffer from autoimmune diseases.

Multiple Sclerosis

Multiple Sclerosis (MS) is at least two to three times more common in women than in men and studies have suggested the female to male rate may be as high as three or four to one. This suggests hormones may play a significant role in determining susceptibility to MS.

In MS, the immune system attacks the myelin, the protective sheath that covers nerve fibers and causes communication problems between your brain and the rest of your body.

A 2019 study showed that a ketogenic diet is safe, feasible and well tolerated in subjects with relapsing multiple sclerosis. It is associated with improved fatigue and depression (Brenton).

An earlier study provided evidence the ketogenic diet could improve mitochondrial function and discussed the potential of the ketogenic diet in treating progressive MS (Storoni). The concept being explored is that the ketogenic diet appears to benefit the body at the cellular level by increasing the amount of nutrients available to the cells while reducing oxidative stress and increasing antioxidant levels in the blood. This research also referred to the potential role of mitochondrial dysfunction in neurodegeneration. The ketogenic diet enhances mitochondrial function.

There is research suggesting MS may impair the brain's ability to use glucose (Regenold). The ketogenic diet converts glucose into ketones as an alternative fuel source for the brain. There's evidence in mice models that by providing an alternative fuel source, the ketogenic diet may be able to help with the neurodegenerative aspect of MS (Kim, Storoni).

It is important that if you are going to try the carnivore diet for your MS, you work with a medical professional who can monitor your progress.

Lupus

Lupus affects women nine times more often than men. It's estimated 1.5 million Americans have lupus. About 9 out of 10 diagnosed are women aged 15 to 44. African American women are three times more likely to get lupus than white women. Lupus is also more common in Hispanic, Asian and Native American women.

Lupus can attack any part of the body. Systemic lupus erythematosus (SLE) is the most common type of lupus. Common symptoms include fatigue, hair loss, sun sensitivity, painful and swollen joints, unexplained fever, skin rashes, and kidney problems.

Studies have shown lupus activates inflammasome NLRP3 which cause inflammation in the body (Zhang). The inflammation leads to debilitating pain. The ketone beta-hydroxybutyrate (BHB) produced when you are in ketosis reduces this inflammation by inhibiting the NLRP3 (Youm). Eating a ketogenic diet and being in ketosis provides a flood of anti-inflammatory ketones.

To date, no studies have been done on the ketogenic diet and lupus, however, the linkage of reduction of inflammation and ketogenic diet is a good beginning. Because it is also successful in helping with weight loss, improving heart and brain health, and improving gut health, it should be beneficial to those with lupus. The carnivore diet may be a good fit for a person with lupus to consider in partnership with a medical professional.

Rheumatoid Arthritis (RA)

Rheumatoid arthritis (RA) means your immune system attacks the healthy cells in your body causing inflammation mainly in the joints. New cases of RA are typically two to three times higher in women than men. The inflammation causes swelling and ultimately thickening of the tissues lining your joints. It can lead to cartilage and bone damage and it is incredibly painful.

People with RA often have low levels of the antioxidant glutathione (Hassan).   This antioxidant is a key player in your immune system. Glutathione is a major
 element in warding off free radicals and protecting your body from oxidative stress. When oxidation in your body isn't balanced with an antioxidant like glutathione, inflammation can take over.   An animal study showed that the ketogenic diet increases glutathione and protects mitochondrial DNA against oxidative damage (Jarrett).

The carnivore diet can provide an anti-inflammatory benefit and enhanced antioxidant activity.   In addition, as with other autoimmune diseases, the carnivore diet can provide a healthier diet with weight loss, improved heart and brain health, and gut health.   The diet should be undertaken in conjunction with a medical professional.

Bipolar Disorder

Bipolar disorder is a serious medical condition that causes extreme swings in a person's mood, energy, and ability to function. These mood changes are called manic and depressive episodes, and are not the typical ups and downs that everyone goes through from time to time. There are different types of bipolar disorder, the two more common being bipolar I and bipolar II.

Women and men are equally likely to have bipolar I disorder, but women are more likely to have bipolar II disorder and may experience more rapid cycling between highs and lows (Freeman).

Women with bipolar are more likely than men with bipolar to have other physical and mental health conditions, including problems with alcohol use, depression caused by bipolar disorder, thyroid disease, obesity caused by medicines used to treat bipolar disorder, and migraine headaches (Freeman).

Changing hormones during the menstrual cycle and menopause can also effect how severe a woman's bipolar disorder is, but they do not cause bipolar disorder (Sit). Women who have bipolar disorder are at risk for experiencing an episode after giving birth, especially a depressive episode (Patchiorotti). Women who experience a depressive or manic episode are also more likely to have episodes after other pregnancies. Women with bipolar disorder are at high risk of developing postpartum psychosis, which is a medical emergency.

Some aspects of the illness, such as illness severity, may be worse for women than for men (Arnold). Panic disorder may be more common (Saunders) while mixed episodes, depressive episodes (Robb) and rapid cycling may occur more frequently for women (Robb, Erol).

Reproductive-cycle events such as menstrual cycles, (Teatero) pregnancy, the postpartum period, (Viquera) and menopause (Chen (a)) may be marked by increased mood disturbances for women with bipolar disorder, with 77% of women reporting worsening of mood at any of those times (Perich).

Other studies have also noted that 20% of women with bipolar disorder are at increased risk of mood episodes during menopause (Blehar). It has been reported that midlife women with major depression and symptomatic menopausal transition have an increased risk of subsequent bipolar disorder compared to those with major depression alone (Chen (a)).

Bipolar disorder and epilepsy share a number of clinical biochemical and physiologic features. Both conditions cycle, both are risk factors for each other, and anticonvulsant drugs used in epilepsy have been found to be effective in helping to manage bipolar illness (www.dietdoctor.com/low-carb/mental-health). Electroconvulsive therapy (ECT) increases seizure threshold, making it more difficult to trigger an attack, and is effective for treating both mania and depression. (Perugi, Weiner).

Epilepsy and bipolar disorder also share many other features, including similar neurotransmitter imbalances such as serotonin, norepinephrine, GABA and glutamate, alterations in sodium and calcium distribution, and changes in chemical messenger activity (www.diagnosisdiet.com/bipolar-disorder-and-low-carb-diets/).

The ketogenic diet was originally introduced as a therapy for epilepsy in 1923 and was used with very good results until medication replaced it. Extensive studies have since shown the ketogenic diet has a positive outcome of treating epileptic seizures (Boison, Williams), and is still recommended today.

In 2013, two women with type II bipolar disorder were able to maintain ketosis for prolonged periods of time (2 and 3 years). Both experienced mood stabilization that exceeded that achieved with medication; experienced a significant subjective improvement that was distinctly related to ketosis, and tolerated the diet well with no significant adverse effects (Phelps).

While further studies need to be done in the area of ketogenic diets and bipolar disorder, it is clear that a ketogenic diet like the carnivore diet could be beneficial to a person with bipolar disorder. There are many examples of people in the carnivore community who have bipolar disorder who have benefited from the carnivore diet. It is important that any changes to one's medications be done in conjunction with a medical professional over an extended period of time.

Depression

Depression is a mood disorder that causes a persistent feeling of sadness and loss of interest. It affects how you feel, think and behave, and can lead to a variety of emotional and physical problems.

The "serotonin hypothesis" of depression proposes that diminished serotonin pathways play a causal role in depression. Serotonin is produced in the digestive tract. It's formed from the amino acid tryptophan. The body can't manufacture tryptophan, so we need to get it from our diet.

If you've been on a poor diet, you are probably deficient in tryptophan and therefore may have low serotonin levels. Foods highest in protein tend to have the highest levels of tryptophan. These include milk, cheese, red meat, eggs, fatty fish and poultry. A serving of poultry supplies about half your recommended daily allowance (RDA) of tryptophan.

L-glutamin is an amino acid made by the body from glutamate that plays a part in brain development and function. Those with depression may have lower levels of glutamine. You can easily get it naturally from foods like beef, chicken, bone broth, and wild fish.

Studies have shown ketones, when administered in the form of endogenous ketones (supplements) in controlled doses, produce blood levels comparable to those achieved by the most rigorous keto diet (Hashim).

Because strict adherence to a keto diet is often difficult for those experiencing psychiatric issues, the administration of endogenous ketone supplements including medium chain triglycerides (MCTs), ketone salts, and ketone esters presents a strategy to circumvent dietary restriction to rapidly induce and sustain nutritional ketosis (Poff, Ari, D'Agostino). However, the exact metabolic effects of exogenous ketones are unknown.

There are no guidelines for using endogenous ketones for the treatment of mood disorders. The research shows, however, that ketones do have an impact. The endogenous ketones are considered to be favored in instances where strict adherence to a ketogenic diet is not sustainable. These levels can also be attained by going on the carnivore diet and reaching ketosis.

In a 2017 study, three men took part in three randomized metabolic studies of drinks containing a ketone ester or ketone salts. Both ketone drinks lowered blood glucose. It was concluded that exogenous ketones are a practical efficacious way to achieve ketosis (Stubbs).

Studies done on rats have shown the production of ketones to be an effective way to manage anxiety (Hollis, Yamanashi). Another rat study concluded the keto diet may have antidepressant properties (Murphy).

It's important if you decide to go on a carnivore diet, or make any changes in your depression medications, you do so in conjunction with a medical professional.

Diabetes

Diabetes is a disease in which blood sugar (glucose) levels in your body are too high. It can cause serious health problems including heart attack and stroke, blindness, problems during pregnancy and kidney failure. About 15 million, or about one out of every nine adult women in the United States have diabetes.

There are three types of diabetes: type 1, type 2 and gestational. In type 1, your body does not make enough insulin, so you have to take insulin every day. Type 2 diabetes is the most common form. With type 2 diabetes, your body doesn't make enough insulin or is not able to use its own insulin correctly. When this happens, blood glucose rises and can get out of control. Gestational diabetes happens only during pregnancy and can cause problems for both the mother and the baby. Having diabetes during pregnancy raises your risk for diabetes 2 later on.

Diabetes affects women and men differently. Compared with men, women have a higher rate of heart disease. It's the number one complication of diabetes. Women have lower rates of survival and a poorer quality of life after a heart attack. They have a higher risk of blindness.

Women with diabetes have a higher risk of depression. Depression also raises the risk for diabetes in women.

The longer you have type 2 diabetes, the higher your risk for developing serious medical problems. The extra glucose in your blood can damage your nerves and blood vessels. Nerve damage from diabetes can lead to pain or a permanent loss of feeling in your hands, feet and other parts of your body. Blood vessel damage from diabetes can also lead to kidney failure, leg or foot amputation and hearing loss.

Women with diabetes are at higher risk for problems getting pregnant, problems during pregnancy, and repeated urinary and vaginal infections. After menopause, women are at higher risk for weight gain, especially more weight around the waist, which raises the risk for type 2 diabetes.

A 2017 study showed individuals with type 2 diabetes improved their glycemic control and lost more weight on a ketogenic diet then on a conventional low fat diabetes diet. (Saslow). In 2018, research found the ketogenic diet to be an effective alternative that relies less on medication and may even be a preferable option when medications are not available (Westman).

Although ketogenic diets are popular among clinicians and patients, the appropriateness of reducing carbohydrate intake in obese patients and patients with diabetes is still debated. However, a 2019 study reviewed the possible role of ketogenic diets in the pathogenesis and management of type 2 diabetes and obesity and found the ketogenic diet can be an effective option (Bolla).

People who have gone on the carnivore diet say it has stabilized their blood sugar. If a person is only eating meat and animal products, they are not taking in glucose. Therefore the blood glucose levels are not going to be affected. The carnivore diet can be a good alternative for a person with diabetes 2.

Heart Disease

The bad news is that heart disease is the leading cause of death for women in the United States (Westerman). And women are more likely to die from their heart attacks than men.

The good news is the majority of recent studies amply demonstrate that the reduction of carbohydrates to levels that induce ketosis can lead to significant benefits in lipid profiles (Brehm, Volek(c)). You can improve your chances of not dying from a heart attack through a ketogenic diet. However, if you currently suffer from heart, kidney or lung disease, the carnivore diet should only be undertaken under medical supervision.

A concern for eating red meat and heart disease has been raised with several recent studies (Wang(a), Heianza). The concern is that elevated levels of tri methyamineN-oxide (TMAO) via gut bacteria are caused by the ingestion of red meat. TMAO is believed to be produced when gut bacteria digest carnitine and choline, nutrients available in red meat, liver and other animal products such as eggs.

However, TMAO is also produced in abundance in fish (Landfold). The authors cite a study which questions the paradox of fish containing considerable amounts of TMAO, yet are generally accepted as cardio protective (Cho). The study suggests the consumption of fish yields substantially greater increases in circulating TMAO than eggs or beef. The conclusion of the study is that TMAO production is a function of individual differences in the gut biome.

Dr. Paul Saladino, explained TMOA in terms of insulin resistance in a August 2019 appearance on a Youtube HVMN presentation hosted by Geoffery Woo (https://www.youtube.com/watch?v=486VfDMEiwY&t=75s).   He related that formation of TMAO in the liver is under the control of an enzyme called FMO3 (flavin-containing monooxygenase-3).   That enzyme is under the control of insulin.   People who are insulin resistant have higher levels of insulin and make more FMO3.   It follows that those who are insulin resistant would have a higher level of TMAO.

Is getting a high level of TMAO from insulin resistance the same as getting a high level from choline and carnitine, the precursors of TMOA? Dr. Saladino answers no.   He states that in all probability it is not that TMAO causes cardiovascular disease, it's that insulin resistance associated with cardiovascular disease probably causes high TMOA. We need choline and carnitine in our bodies, and to limit them out of fear for TMAO is to move the health of the population in a clearly negative direction.

A 2002 study examined the effects of a six-week ketogenic diet and results suggested a ketogenic diet does not have a deleterious effect on cardiovascular risk profile (Sharman). Noting very low carbohydrate (ketogenic) diets are popular but controversial, a 2005 study reviewed summarized studies that had examined the effects of very low carbohydrate (ketogenic) diets on lipoproteins and related risk factors for cardiovascular disease. Prospective studies indicate that very low carbohydrate (ketogenic) diets improve lipoprotein profile independently of weight loss. They also improve pro inflammatory markers when associated with weight loss (Volek(d)).

Low carbohydrate, ketogenic diets have a positive effect on cardiovascular disease.

Leaky Gut

Leaky gut, or intestinal permeability, is a condition in which the lining of the small intestine becomes damaged, causing undigested food particles, toxic waste products, and bacteria to leak through the intestines and flood the bloodstream. Mainstream medicine has largely dismissed the theory of illnesses being linked to a "leaky gut" as "pseudo-science."

But recent research is confirming that a breakdown of the gut barrier can occur (Fasano (a)(b)). Over the last decade a number of academic institutions from around the world have been showing that an increase in intestinal permeability is a common feature of a number of autoimmune and chronic disease conditions (Konig, Bischoff).

In order to be healthy, your intestine absorbs nutrients and energy for use by the body, but keeps out microbes, antigens and other disease-causing agents. The theory is that increased permeability allows unwanted substances to cross the intestinal barrier, triggering inflammation and a dysfunctional immune response.

The gastrointestinal (GI) tract has its own nervous system, known as the enteric nervous system (ENS). The ENS is a collection of 500 million neurons and is in every part of your gut, from the esophagus, clear down to the end. Scientists have recently figured out how it works (Spencer); the gut communicates with the central nervous system via the vagus nerve.

Ninety percent of the serotonin our body makes is produced in the GI tract, and half of of the dopamine is made there too. We think that anxiety and depression contribute to gut problems. But studies show it may be the other way around. Researchers are finding evidence that irritation in the gastrointestinal system may send signals to the central nervous system that trigger mood changes. These messages are sent *to* the brain rather than being received *from* it. This could be why a high-than-normal percentage of people with irritable bowel syndrome (IBS) and functional bowel problems develop depression and anxiety. It becomes even more likely if a person suffers from leaky gut.

When it comes to gut health, eating a carnivore diet can make your gut healthier in several ways. By not eating sugars or refined carbohydrates, you're not feeding unwanted bacteria in the gut. Two main foods associated with a weak gut are grains and beans; gluten, lectins and oxalates also contribute to gut lining damage. Eating a carnivore diet removes exposure to GMO foods, pesticides or antibiotics in plants that can quickly devastate the balance of gut bacteria.

Elimination of them in the carnivore diet creates a stronger gut lining. And by consuming the recommended amount of animal products in a day, you provide yourself with 100% - 300% of vitamins important for your health.

There are an increasing number of doctors recommending the ketogenic diet to treat a wide variety of medical conditions. One clinic, Paleomedicina in Zalaszentgrot, Hungary, treats a wide array of autoimmune conditions such as type 1 and type 2 diabetes, mental health conditions, and even cancer.

Their protocol follows what the clinic believes the early modern humans evolved to eat. The diet consists of a paleo-carnivore diet of red meats and organ meats. Since 2013, the clinic has treated more than 10,000 patients. They've had excellent results in the reversal of Crohn's disease, a chronic inflammatory bowel disease (IBD) characterized by inflammation of the GI tract (Toth).

They say their research suggests a key mechanism of the diet is its positive function of the intestine, healing and reversing intestinal permeability, or leaky gut.(http://www.dietdoctor.com/low-carb/carnivore#paleomedicina)

Migraines

Of the more than 39 million American sufferers of migraine headaches, 28 million are women. Migraine is one of the leading serious health problems affecting women. Women experience migraine differently than men. Women report episodic pain, often for a longer duration, and chronic pain more frequently than men More severe and more frequent migraine attacks often result from changes in estrogen levels.

Women suffer from migraine three times as often as men in the U.S., and during the reproductive years, as many as 37% of women suffer. Of those who suffer, 50% have more than one attack each month, and 25% have four or more severe attacks per month. Many women find their migraine symptoms are affected by menstruation, hormonal contraception, pregnancy and menopause. (https://migraineresearchfoundation.org)

A debilitating migraine headache is not just a bad headache. It's a neurological disorder and ultimately affects one's quality of life. A migraine is defined as a recurrent throbbing headache that typically affects one side of the head and is often accompanied by nausea and disturbed vision. There are no current treatment options that do the job well or that are absent of unwanted side effects. It is not fully understood what causes migraines.

Ketones have successfully treated migraines since 500 AD. The keto diet became popular nearly a century ago (Wheless) when it was used to treat epilepsy.

Ketones block high concentrations of glutamate found in both migraine and epilepsy sufferers (Maalouf(b)).   Anti-seizure medications that block glutamate have been used to treat both migraine and epilepsy sufferers (Rogawski). A 2013 study found the ketogenic diet reduced migraines in 90% of patients (DiLorenzo).

Obesity may increase migraine risk by 81% (Recober). Ketones reduce hunger as well as glucose and insulin problems and promote weight loss (Paoli). Oxidative stress, a disturbance in the balance between the production of free radicals and antioxidant defenses, has been tied to all migraine triggers (Borkum, Gupta). Ketones not only block excess glutamate, but also reduce total levels of oxidative stress (Maalouf (b), Milder Rhyu). This suggests that ketones prevent migraine and may even prevent the root cause of migraines.

Vulvodynia

A diet low in oxalates has been suggested as a treatment for women who experience unexplained pain in the area of the vulva, or vulvodynia. By virtue of eliminating plants and replacing them with high protein meat and animal products, the carnivore diet can be used as a treatment.

A woman's illness, vulvodynia is the term used to explain the condition experienced by women who have the sensation of vulval burning and soreness in the absence of any obvious skin condition or infection, according to the Vulval Pain Society (www.vulvalpainsociety.org). This condition is usually a consequence of irritation or hypersensitivity of the nerve fibers in the vulval skin. This type of pain can occur even when the area is not touched. It is compared to the pain of shingles.

The pain can range from mild discomfort to a severe constant pain which can even prevent you from sitting down comfortably. There are good days and bad days. Itching is not usually a feature of the condition. The pain is not always restricted to the vulval area, but can include the inside of the thighs, upper legs and around the anus and uretha.

The association of oxalates and vulval pain was highlighted in an article in an American medical journal in 1991 where a woman with vulvodynia was found to have abnormally high levels of oxalate in her urine. She was treated with a combination of a low-oxalate diet and the use of a food supplement called calcium citrate which removes the oxalate from the body. Following treatment, her symptoms resolved as her urine oxalate levels fell. This is the only reference in the literature which shows the low-oxalate diet is a beneficial treatment; however, it is widely used in the United States as a treatment for vulvodynia. The diet may be supplemented with the use of oral calcium citrate.

While there are no studies which prove a relationship between oxalates and vulvodynia, the carnival diet which contains no oxalates, along with calcium citrate, may benefit women with vulval pain.

Susan Owens, a leader in the investigation of oxalates and their effects, conducts Facebook and Yahoo Groups called Trying Low Oxalates which carry information on the reduction of Oxalates for health benefits.

Conclusion

The carnivore diet is a powerful healing ketogenic diet for women. It's a long term way of life. It provides a high nutrient, low toxin, bioavailable form of eating that is totally different from the standard American diet.

Although both are ketogenic, the difference between a keto diet and the carnivore diet is the carnivore diet excludes all plants, fruits, vegetables, grains, nuts and seeds. It also contains a higher level of protein.

There are numerous ways to accomplish the carnivore diet. It can be done with a wide variety of animal products, including beef, pork, chicken, lamb, fish, seafood, hard cheese, butter and eggs. It can be just meat, water and salt. It can include offal, or animal organs, or not.

It requires decisions by each individual as to whether they need to include supplemental vitamins based on what they are eating and whether it is providing them with enough nutrients. This is accomplished by paying attention to your own body and working with a medical professional if you have a concern.

When you begin the carnivore diet, if you have been on a plant-based diet, be aware of the effects anti-nutrient withdrawal may have on your body and slowly ease into it. You may also experience keto flu and suffer the loss of electrolytes in the first couple weeks of the diet due to loss of water. Be sure to compensate by adding salt to your food. You may need to supplement calcium, magnesium and potassium during the adaptation portion of the carnivore diet.

Remember fats are your friend and help absorb minerals and vitamins. You have to eat fat to lose fat—good saturated fats are found in red meat, whole-milk dairy foods, cheese, eggs, fatty fish and poultry. It's not the fats and cholesterol, it is carbohydrates and sugars that make a negative impact on one's lipid profile and risk factors.

Low fiber isn't associated with constipation, and fiber isn't necessary for nutrients and digestive health. That's a real shocker, but there's lots of scientific research to prove it. You'll probably experience a change in bowel habits one way or the other when first beginning the carnivore diet, but this will calm down after a couple of days to a week as your body adjusts to this new way of eating.

One of the biggest hurdles to get over with the carnivore diet is the idea that we can get our vitamins from meat. Meat!! Let's put this into perspective. We can get our vitamins if we eat a well rounded variety of animal products including offal, or organ meat, fish and seafood. Because we no longer consume toxic plant-based foods, we absorb food nutrients better and make better use of our vitamins and minerals. If we don't eat a well rounded variety of animal products, it is up to each of us to make the decision as to whether to supplement our diet with vitamins and minerals. Many choose to take a supplemental vitamin and/or additional magnesium, potassium, and calcium. Some take vitamin C. It is up to the individual to monitor their body and make good informed decisions about their own health.

Intermittent fasting is a way of scheduling your meals to provide your body with a fasting state on a regular basis. It can have powerful effects on your body and has been a missing link in women's health. Your cells initiate a cellular repair process with intermittent fasting. There are a myriad of health benefits that, coupled with the carnivore diet, can contribute to a long, healthy life

Exercise is a choice. Of course, it's good for you! But, you may choose to just concentrate on the carnivore diet for the first month. And when you add exercise, it may just be walking. Or you may feel you can do more and you can! It's up to you! Light activity or resistance training are both good options for exercise. But the carnivore diet is not believed to be compatible with competitive or strenuous exercise, although it may be part of an overall strategy.

The carnivore diet affects women through ketosis. It affects women's hormones, particularly insulin, cortisol, thyroid, estrogen, progesterone and testosterone. Women with insulin resistance are helped with a ketogenic diet. Women with polycystic ovarian syndrome (PCOS) have insulin resistance and glucose intolerance, and the ketogenic carnivore diet can be helpful in combating this disease.

Metabolic syndrome is a cluster of symptoms that appear together which increase your risk of heart disease, stroke and type 2 diabetes. These conditions include increased blood pressure, high blood sugar, excess body fat around the waist and abnormal cholesterol or triglyceride levels. Metabolic syndrome is closely linked to insulin resistance, as well as overweight or obesity and inactivity.

More than two in three women in the United States are overweight or obese. That extra weight leads to many diseases that affect women, such as heart disease, diabetes and many cancers. Studies have shown the ketogenic diet significantly reduces body weight, glucose and cholesterol levels.

Your thyroid gland produces thyroid hormone which controls many activities in your body, including affecting ovulation, your metabolism and your heart. A ketogenic diet can decrease T3 hormone, but a lowered T3 isn't the same thing as hypothyroidism. When only T3 is decreased, your thyroid is considered to be normal.

Cortisol is called the stress hormone in the body. Control your stress and you'll control your cortisol! Starting a ketogenic diet and removing carbohydrates from your diet forces your body to deal with carbohydrate withdrawal, which is stressful. And your cortisol production may increase. But once your body adapts, usually within three to four weeks, your cortisol levels will return to normal.

Your ovaries produce estrogen, progesterone, and testosterone. Having too much fat on your body increases your estrogen levels. But, biologically, we women are programmed to stock up on fat for perceived future pregnancies. Our bodies try to store fat at every chance they get. And that increases our estrogen production. But weight loss means lower estrogen production.

If you've had irregular periods, the carnivore diet can help normalize them. Many premenstrual symptoms (PMS) improve. Often the underlying cause of PMS is estrogen dominance caused by having too much estrogen and not enough progesterone. One of the causes of estrogen dominance is a diet high in sugar and refined carbohydrates. This improves with a carnivore diet.

The estrogens provide brain protective actions and their loss during aging and natural or surgical menopause is associated with dysfunction, age related disorders and signs of Alzheimer's. An emerging strategy to compensate for deteriorating brain energy is the use of the brain's alternative source to glucose—ketones.

It is thought ketogenic interventions in the form of a ketogenic diet or exogenous ketones may delay Alzheimer's disease. Studies have shown that attempting to treat cognitive deficit early in Alzheier's disease using ketogenic interventions in clinical
 trials is safe, ethical and scientifically well-founded.

In menopause, we've lost the protection of estrogen and our gut biome goes through a major shift. This causes a reduction in neurotransmitter production, ultimately leading to chronic inflammation, a slower metabolism and poor sleep. We get hit with belly fat, brain fog, memory loss, headaches, low libido, mood swings and hot flashes. Ketones produced from a ketogenic diet such as the carnivore diet give us some relief.

The health of your immune system dictates the health of every cell in your body. In the case of autoimmune diseases, your immune system starts to mistake healthy cell tissues in your body as outside invaders. Examples are Hashimoto's and Graves' thyroiditis, rheumatoid arthritis, lupus, Chrohn's disease, multiple sclerosis, and type 1 and type 2 diabetes.

In multiple sclerosis, the immune system attacks the myelin. Studies show the ketogenic diet benefits the body at the cellular level, has improved mitochondrial function, reduced oxidative stress, and is well tolerated in subjects.

Lupus affects 1.5 million women and 90% are of child bearing age. It causes inflammation leading to debilitating pain. Eating a ketogenic diet provides anti-inflammatory ketones.

Rheumatoid arthritis (RA) means your immune system attacks the healthy cells in your body causing inflammation mainly in the joints. People with RA often have low levels of the antioxidant glutathione, which is a key player in your immune system. Glutathione is a major element in warding off free radicals and protecting your body from oxidative stress. When oxidation in your body isn't balanced with an antioxidant like glutathione, inflammation can take over. An animal study showed that the ketogenic diet increases glutathione and protects mitochondrial DNA against oxidative damage (Jarrett). The carnivore diet can provide an anti-inflammatory benefit and enhanced antioxidant activity.

Bipolar disorder is a serious medical condition that causes extreme swings in a person's mood, energy, and ability to function. Changing hormones during the menstrual cycle and menopause can affect how severe a woman's bipolar disorder is. Bipolar disorder and epilepsy share a number of clinical biochemical and physiologic features. The ketogenic diet was originally introduced as a therapy for epilepsy in 1923 and was used with very good results. It is still recommended today. It is clear that a ketogenic diet like the carnivore diet could be beneficial to a person with bipolar disorder. There are many examples of people in the carnivore community who have bipolar disorder who have benefited from the carnivore diet.

Depression is a mood disorder that causes a persistent feeling of sadness and loss of interest. The "serotonin hypothesis" of depression proposes that diminished serotonin pathways play a causal role in depression Serotonin is produced in the digestive tract from tryptophan. The body can't manufacture tryptophan, so we need to get it from our diet. Foods containing tryptophan are red meat, whole milk dairy foods, cheese, eggs, fatty fish and poultry—foods from the carnivore diet.

Those with depression are also low in L-glutamin, an amino acid made by the body from glutamate that plays a part in brain development and functions. You can easily get it from foods like beef, chicken, bone broth and wild fish, again, carnivore diet foods. Studies have shown that ketones when administered in the form of endogenous ketones (supplements) in controlled doses, produce blood levels comparable to those achieved by the most rigorous keto diet.

Diabetes is a disease in which blood sugar (glucose) levels in your body are too high. It can cause serious health problems including heart attack and stroke, blindness, problems during pregnancy and kidney failure. Women with diabetes have a higher rate of heart disease than men with diabetes. And they have a lower rate of survival. Numerous studies have found the ketogenic diet to be an effective and even preferable alternative to a conventional low fat diabetes diet. Diabetics who have gone on the carnivore diet say it has stabilized their blood sugar. The carnivore diet can be a good alternative for a person with diabetes 2.

Heart disease is the leading cause of death for women in the United States. However, recent studies amply demonstrate that you can improve your chances of not dying from a heart attack through a ketogenic diet. If you suffer from heart, kidney or lung disease, the carnivore diet should only be undertaken under medical supervision.

Of the more than 39 million American sufferers of migraine headaches, 28 million are women.   A debilitating migraine headache is not just a bad headache. It's a neurological disorder and ultimately affects one's quality of life The carnivore diet can be used to reduce migraines.   Ketones not only prevent migraine headaches, but may even prevent the root cause of them.

Vulvodynia is a condition experienced by women who have the sensation of vulval burning and soreness in the absence of any obvious skin condition or infection.   It is compared to the pain of shingles. A diet low in oxalates has been suggested as a treatment for women who experience unexplained pain the the area of the vulva. By virtue of eliminating plants and replacing them with high protein meat and animal products, the carnivore diet can be used as a treatment.

The carnivore diet is a diet that works for many people under many circumstances. It is a long term healthy way of eating that depends on each individual making good choices for themselves. My hope is that this book will guide you in those choices.

Come visit my blog at
www.claudiadrake.org

Looking for a good support group?
Check out "Women Carnivore Tribe" on Facebook

Glossary

Beta-hydroxybutyrate (BHB):
One of the three ketones produced and burned in our cells in ketosis.

Carnivore Diet:
A healing, ketogenic diet which excludes plants.

Electrolytes:
Minerals involved in many essential processes in your body.

Exogenous Ketones:
Exogenous ketones come from an external source not produced in the body. They are consumed as supplements.

Glucose:
A simple sugar which is an energy source.

Glycogen:
A substance deposited in bodily tissues as a store of carbohydrates; a storage form of glucose.

Keto Diet:
A high fat, moderate protein, low-carbohydrate diet that allows your body to burn ketones. It usually consists of meat, fish, seafood, nuts, seeds, beans, veggies and some berries.

Ketogenic Diet:
A diet where a state of burning fat for energy is entered into which produces ketones.

Ketone:
Substance produced from burning fat through a low-carb diet or fasting, used as a source of energy in your body.

Ketosis:
The process of burning fat for energy; the presence of ketones in the body.

Nose-to-tail:
A philosophy of eating and cooking that involves using every possible part of an animal, e.g., liver, heart, tongue, hooves, ears, bone marrow, etc.

Offal:
The internal organs of an animal, e.g., heart and liver, etc.

APPENDIX A
Why Many Carnivores Don't Use Supplements

This information is taken from *The Ultimate Guide to the Carnivore Diet"* by L. Amber O'Hearn and Raphael Sirtoli, Chapter 4, Section 3. Antinutrients and Metabolic Change. It has been modified for brevity and I have added my own comments, which are highlighted in italics. The original can be found at <u>http://nutrita.app/guide-to-the-carnivore-diet</u>

O'Hearn and Sirtoli explain that plants contain "anti-nutrients," factors that make food less nutritious. It's been shown that the consumption of grains, nuts, beans and other seeds interfere with the absorption of certain minerals, particularly zinc (Lonnerdahl), but also others including calcium, magnesium, chromium, iron and manganese. This effect is largely due to phytates, anti-nutrients found in the seeds of plants. It's thought to be a protective mechanism for plant reproduction.

In figuring out our Recommended Daily Allowance (RDA) of vitamins and minerals, our government established guidelines based on a high carbohydrate, grain based diet. This means that RDAs for these minerals are greatly overestimated for someone who isn't eating the refined carbs, sugar, vegetables, grains, nuts and seeds of the standard American diet.

The other reason that many of the RDAs are likely to be higher than what we need on a carnivore diet is that shortly after we begin the diet, we begin producing ketones. We get our energy from fat and ketones, not glucose. Much of our requirement for micronutrients is because they are used in chemical processes for producing energy in a way that is different from those on the standard American diet.

For example, levels of the thyroid hormone, T3, depend on how much glucose you use for energy. So if you are using fat for energy, you make less T3. Iodine is used to make T3, so the need for iodine strongly depends on how much glucose you need for energy and should be expected to be lower on a carnivore diet (Kopp).

Since a person on a carnivore diet could very possibly be expected to use less iodine, it seems likely they could require less of other nutrients than the RDA lists. The problem is we don't know how much because no tests or research have been done as of yet.

O'Hearn and Sirtoli go on to consider the micronutrients that people are often concerned about when considering a carnivore diet—the electrolytes potassium, magnesium, and vitamin C.

In adapting to any ketogenic diet, there is an initial stage of water loss that can lead to temporary losses in potassium, sodium and magnesium. For this reason, it is wise to replace these during the adaptation phase. Potassium is a mineral that is abundant in the body. It's necessary for life, and meat contains potassium.

The Institute of Medicine (IOM) determines RDA and publishes documents explaining how they came up with them. In the chapter on potassium, they explain there was insufficient information to make an RDA for potassium, so the RDA was hard to determine (Potassium). They couldn't find enough experiments to prove a particular amount would reduce the effects they are concerned about. Those effects were high blood pressure, kidney stones and possible bone loss. Instead they determined adequate intake based in large part on epidemiological studies that correlated intakes with these issues in a high carb, plant based population (Potassium).

One factor they did cite as affecting potassium balance was fiber intake, with more fiber resulting in more potassium passing through undigested. *This potassium wouldn't have been absorbed and would have been wasted. A carnivore eats no fiber as there is no fiber in meat or animal products, and would absorb a higher amount of the potassium.*

Another factor they cited was sodium intake. Basically, the more salt you consume, the more potassium you need to balance it. So if you add salt to your carnivore diet, as most carnivores do, you may be more likely to have inadequate potassium than a carnivore who doesn't.

Researcher Stephen Phinney has pointed out that preserving lean mass requires adequate potassium. In his review "Ketogenic Diets and Physical Performance," he reported on male cyclists in a metabolic ward on a ketogenic diet (Phinney). Through a combination of meat and supplements the subjects were taking 2 to 3 g of potassium a day. Although there were some initial losses during adaptation, after four weeks, potassium levels stabilized. This is less than the RDA by almost half.

Beef and pork contain 300 to 400 mg of potassium per 100 g, or about 3.5 oz a serving. Roughly, you'd need about 1.5 to 2 pounds, or 0.7 to 1 kg of meat a day to reach the level of potassium in that experiment. Most carnivores do eat this amount of meat a day *at a minimum.* Moreover, most carnivores are not losing lean mass, which would be expected with a potassium deficiency.

Magnesium absorption is affected by fiber and by phytates. The first two sections in the IOMs chapter on magnesium requirements talks about how magnesium absorption is very negatively affected by fiber, phytates and inadequate levels of protein (Magnesium). Since none of these are a concern on the carnivore diet, we should expect that our need for magnesium intake is considerably less than average.

And again, there was not a lot of data available to examine what the real need was. Most of the experiments used to determine adequate levels were simply the levels found in self-selected control diets in experiments designed to deliberately cause magnesium depletion. Because of these experiments, the current recommended RDA for magnesium is largely based on the amount you would need for a typical typical western diet with a lot of fiber or high oxalate plants in it, or not enough protein.

Many people in the general population test low for magnesium blood levels (Whang). Some researchers are calling for raising the reference range, largely because more people at the bottom half of the range have been found to have symptoms of metabolic syndrome (Costello).

But do people on a carnivore diet have low levels of magnesium? In a study of 50 patients following a paleo-carnivore diet, only one person was below reference range, and even then, just barely (Clemons). *It should be noted these participants were being treated for ailments where they probably had low levels of magnesium to begin with and their meals included extensive amounts of offal (organ meats) such as liver, heart, brain, etc.*

Even if people on a carnivore diet did have lower levels of magnesium, would that put them at risk for metabolic syndrome? The answer is believed to be no, given that low carbohydrate diets reliably reduce markers of metabolic syndrome. In light of this, it seems more likely that carnivorous dieters would have normal levels of magnesium, despite lower intake.

If you are concerned about magnesium levels, you can have your blood levels checked and see where you are in the range. Another way to tell is by calcium and potassium levels. At moderate levels of deficiency, both calcium and potassium will often be low (Rude, Huang).

"Early signs of a serious deficiency would result in serious symptoms, like loss of appetite, nausea, vomiting, fatigue and weakness. . . As magnesium deficiency worsens, numbness, tingling, muscle contractions and cramps, seizures, personality changes, abnormal heart beat and coronary spasms can occur." (Jahnen-Dechnen)

Vitamin C is another nutrient that is hard to meet the RDA on meat alone. Despite that, meat has been known since the times of early Arctic explorers specifically for its ability to cure scurvy, the disease that results from lack of vitamin C.

Adding to the confusion, the USDA data base lists beef, pork and bone marrow as having no vitamin C, even though this isn't technically true (O'Hearn, Metzner). The amount of vitamin C in those meats is, in fact, probably enough to combat scurvy if it's eaten in the high amounts most carnivores do, and if it's not overcooked, as cooking destroys vitamin C. Anecdotally, many long term carnivores have gone years without supplemental vitamin C and show no signs of scurvy, which take only a couple of months to appear.

But the RDA for vitamin C is set way higher than the amount needed to prevent scurvy. One reason carnivores aren't concerned is because the remainder of the RDA is based on speculative reasoning about antioxidants. Oxidation is a natural process that happens continuously in the body It's a matter of balance. When oxidation is offset by anti-oxidation, life proceeds normally. It is when oxidation gets out of proportion that disease happens.

Vitamin C is an antioxidant, but it's not the only antioxidant, and it's not even one of the most important ones. The most important ones are the ones we make ourselves, including uric acid and glutathione. There have been animal studies showing that sufficient glutathione prevents vitamin C deficiency by sparing its use (Martennsen). Glutathion may be higher in ketogenic diets since its precursors—the building blocks used to build it—are abundant in meat (Jarret).

O'Hearn and Sirtoli write that the speculation behind the need for extra vitamin C is based largely on the hope that its antioxidant properties might help with heart disease and diabetes, both metabolic diseases. But study results are mixed and inconclusive. The therapeutic effect of a low carb diet on markers of metabolic syndrome diseases greatly outweigh any observed effects of vitamin C on them.

Ironically, one of the greatest drivers of oxidative stress is glucose (Ede). Gucose competes with vitamin C for uptake in cells, meaning that lower blood sugar increases the availability of whatever vitamin C is there (Price). These reasons might explain why we don't so far see any negative health consequences of lower vitamin C intake in carnivores.

Vitamin C helps us form collagen, a crucial component of functional arteries and youthful skin It also helps synthesize L-carnitine, a compound that helps us burn fat by transporting fats into our mitochondria. By eating a carnitine-rich diet, we'll have less need for vitamin C to synthesize carnitine, thus freeing more of it for collagen synthesis and other crucial processes (Strijbis). Animal foods are high in carnitine. This may be one way carnivore diet are vitamin C sparing.

And the best source of vitamin C in meat? Liver, especially chicken liver—*a couple ounces a day would more than take care of nutrient needs for a carnivore.*

Meat is very high in most nutrients and those that are more difficult to get with meat are likely to be needed in lower amounts than generally believed. Given this fact, many carnivores skip supplements. Others take the ones they are concerned about. It's very much a personal choice.

APPENDIX B
Oxalate Research

The following research on oxalates is taken from "Lost Seasonality and Overconsumption of Plants: Risking Oxalate Toxicity," Sally K. Norton, Journal of Evolution and Health, Vol 2, Issue 3, Symposium 2017 (https://jevohealth.com/cgi/viewcontent.cgi?article=1085&context=journal).

Multiple studies show that the typical amounts of oxalate in our diets can easily contribute to oxalate accumulation in non-renal tissues even though the kidneys are healthy and their handling capacity is not exceeded (Heaney, Blumenfrucht, Holmes).

The formation of oxalate micro-crystals is especially common in human thyroid gland and breast tissue (Wang(b), Radi).

A study of 182 normal thyroids found that eighty-five percent of people over age 50 have calcium oxalate crystals in their thyroid gland (Katoh).

Bio-accumulation in humans probably reflects the ubiquity of excessive oxalate in normal diets (Glew, Siener, Chai).

Oxalate has been noted to cause pathological calcification (Salyer, Fishbein, Shavit), weakened bones (Aydin, Maldonado, Brancaccio), and connective tissue (Fielder, Boogaerts, Johnson(b)), tooth mobility (Bimstein, Panis, Lapointe, Hedemark, Moskow), interfere with tissue healing (Mehendale), and promote fibrosis (Salyer, Khan).

Chronic exposure of ionic oxalate alters breast cells, transforming normal breast cells to tumor cells (Castellaro).

Many studies note oxalate-induced central nervous system dysfunction without evidence of micro-crystal accumulation in the brain (Moorhead).

Oxalate toxicity is associated with damage to the function and structure of nerves (Christison, Samarneh, Blyth, Tsai, Auxiliadora-Martins).

Oxalate ions and nano-crystals are increasingly implicated as a cause or aggravator of a wide range of metabolic derangements associated with chronic health issues, (Sun, Mulay, Elferink).

Dramatic increases in calcium-oxalate kidney stones, and functional problems with digestive health (Johnson(a)), health (Johnson(b)), neurotoxicity (Moorhead, Blyth, Lewis, Chen (b), Rahman), sleep, brain function, inflammation (Boogaerts, Adams, Coral, Marconi, Brady, Synmans), chronic pain, autoimmunity, cellular stress, fatigue, arthritis, and connective tissue instability, (Brancaccio, Brady, Reginato, Rubinstein), osteoporosis, and vulnerability to injury are all consistent with increased oxalate toxicity (Shavit, Ermer, Mulay).

References

Adams ND, Carrera GF, Johnson RP, Latorraca R, Lemann J. Calcium-oxalate-crystal-induced bone disease. Am J Kidney Dis Off J Natl Kidney Found 1982;1(5) 294-299

Aksunger FB, Topkaya AE, Akyildiz M, Interleuken-6, C-reactive protein and biochemical parameters during prolonged intermittent fasting. Ann Nutr Metab, 2007; 51(1):88-95

Alirezaei, Mehrdad; Kemball, Christopher C; Flynn, Claudia T; Wood, Malcolm R; Whitten, J. Lindsay; Kiosses, William B. Short-term fasting induces profound neuronal autophagy. Autophagy 2010; Aug 16 6(6):702-710

Alwahab, Ula Abed; Pantalone, Keven M; Burguera, Bartalome. A ketogenic diet may restore fertility in women with polycystic ovary syndrome: A case series. AACE Clinical Case Reports: September/October 2018, Vol 4, No. 5, pp e427-431

Anderson, Pauline. More Evidence Links High Cholesterol to Lower Parkinson's Risk. Medscape Medical News June 14, 2017; https://www.medscape.com/viewarticle/881576

Anson, R. Michael; Gue, Zhihong; deCabo, Rafael; Iyun, Titola; Rios, Michelle; Hagepanos, Adrienne; Ingram, Donald K; Lane, Mark A.; Mattson, Mark P. Intermittent fasting dissociates beneficial effects of dietary restriction on glucose metabolism and neuronal resistance to injury from calorie intake. <u>Proc Natl Acad Sci USA</u> 2003; May 13; 100 (10) 6216-6220

Ari C, Kovac Z, Juhasz G, Murdun C, Goldhagen CR, Koutnik AP, Poff AM, Kesl SL, D'Agostino DP. Exogenous ketone supplements reduce anxiety-related behavior in Sprague-Dawley and Wistar Albino Glaxo/Ryswijk rats. <u>Front Moi Neurosci</u> 2016 Dec 6; 9:137

Arnold IM, Gender differences in bipolar disorder. <u>Psychiatr Clin North Am</u> 2003 Sep 26 (3) 595-620

Assuncao ML, Ferreira HS, dos Santos AF, Cabral CR Jr, Florencio TM. Effects of dietary coconut oil on the biochemical and anthropometric profiles of women presenting abdominal obesity. <u>Lipids</u> 2009 Jul; 44(7): 593-601

Astrup A, Dyerberg J, Elwood P, Hermansen K, Hu FB, Jakobsen MU, Kok FJ, Krauss RM, Lecerf JM, LeGrand P, Nestel P, Riserus U, Sanders T, Sinclair A, Stender S, Tholstrup T, Willett WC. The role of reducing intakes of saturated fat in the prevention of cardiovascular disease: where does the evidence stand in 2010? <u>Am J Clin Nutr</u> 2011 Apr;93(4): 684-8

Auxiliadora-Martins M, Alkmin Teixeira GC, Silva GS da, et al. Severe encephalopathy after ingestion of star fruit juice in a patient with chronic renal failure admitted to the intensive care unit. <u>Heart Lung J Crit Care</u> 2010;39(5): 448-452

Aydin NE, Usta U. Oxalate deposition in tissues. <u>Nephrol Dial Transplant</u> 2004;19(5):1323-1324

Baker LD, Cross DJ, Minoshina S, Belongia D, Watson GS, Craft S. Insulin resistance and Alzheimer-like reductions in regional cerebral glucose metabolism for cognitively normal adults with pre diabetes or early type 2 diabetes. <u>Arch Neurol</u> 2010 Jan;68(1) 51-7

Baranowska, Boguslawa; Wolinska0Witort, Ewa; Bik, Wojciech; Baranowska-Bk, Agnieszka; Martynska, Lidia; Chmielowska, Magdalena. Evaluation of neuroendocrine status in longevity. <u>Neurolbiology of Aging</u>, Volume 28 Issue 5, May 2007, Pages 774-783

Barnosky, Adrienne R; Hoddy, Kristin K; Unterman, Terry G; Varady, Krista A. Intermittent fasting vs daily calorie restriction for type 2 diabetes prevention: a review of human findings. <u>Translational Research</u> Volume 164, Issue 4, October 2014, Pages 302-311

Bimstein E, Wagner M, Nauman RK, Abrams RG, Shapira L. Root surface characteristics of primary teeth from children with prepubertal periodontitis. <u>J Periodontal *1998:69(3):337-347*</u>

Bischoff SC, Barbara G, Buurman Wa, Ockhuizen T, Schulzke J, Serino M, Tilg H, Watson A, Wells JM. Intestinal permeability—a new target for disease prevention and therapy. <u>BMC Gastroenterol</u> 2014 Nov 18;14: 189

Blehar MC, DePaulo JR, Jr, Gershon ES, Reich T, Simpson SG, Nurnberger JR, Jr. Women with bipolar disorder: findings from the NIMH Genegics Initiative Sample. <u>Psychopharmacol Bull</u> 1998; 34(3): 239-43

Blumenfrucht MJ, Cheeks C, Wedeen RP. Multiorgan crystal deposition following intravenous oxalate infusion in rat. <u>J Urol</u> 1986; 135(6): 1274-1279

Blyth AW, and B Meredith, Blyth MW. Poisons: Their Effects and Detection. 4th ed. London, England: Charles Griffin and Company: 1906

Boison D. New insights into the mechanisms of the ketogenic diet. <u>Curr Opin Neurol</u> 2017 Apr, 30(2): 187-192

Bolla, Andrea Mario; Caretto, Amelia; Laurenzi, Andrea; Scavini, Marina; Piemonte, Lorenzo. Low-Carb and Ketogenic Diets in Type 1 and Type 2 Diabetes. <u>Nutrients</u> 2019 May;11(5):962

Bonora E, Kiechl S, Wileit J, Oberhollenzer F, Egger G, Bonndonna RC, Muggeo M, Brunneck study. Caroted atherosclerosis and coronary heart disease in the metabolic syndrome: prospective data from the Brunneck study. <u>Diabetes Care</u> 2003 Apr; 26(4): 1251-7

Boogaerts MA, Hammerschmidt DE, Roelant C, Verwilghen RI, Jacob HS. Mechanisms of vascular damage in gout and oxalosis:

crystal induced, granulocyte mediated, endothelial injury. <u>Thromb Haemost</u> 1983;50(2):576-580

Borkum, Jonathan M. Migraine Triggers and Oxidative Stress: A Narrative Review and Synthesis. <u>Headache</u> 07 December 2015 <u>https://doi.irg.19.1111.head.12625</u>

Brady HR, Fay WP, Meema HE, Rabinovich S, Rapoport A, Oreopoulos DG. Oxalate bone disease—an emerging form of renal osteodystrophy. <u>Int J Artif Organs</u> 1989;12(11): 715-719

Brancaccio D, Poggi A, Ciccarelli C, et al. Bone changes in end-stage oxalises. <u>AJR Am J Roentgenol 1981;136(5): 935-939</u>

Brehm BJ, Seeley RJ, Daniels SR, D'Alessio DA. A randomized trial comparing a very low carbohydrate diet and a calorie-restricted low fat diet on body weight and cardiovascular risk factors in healthy women. <u>J Clin Endocrinol Metab</u> 2003 Apr;88(4): 1617-23

Brenton(a) JN, Banwell B, Bergqvist C, Lehner-Gulotta D, Gampper L, Leytham E, Coleman R, Goldman MD. Pilot Study of a ketogenic diet in relapsing-remitting MS. <u>Neurology</u> July 2019; 6 (4)

Brenton JN, Banwell B, Berggist AC, Lehner-Guiotta D, Gampper I, Leytham F, Coleman R, Goldman MD. Pilot study of a ketogenic diet in relapsing-remitting MS. <u>Neurol Neuroimmunol Neuroinflamm</u> 2019 Apr 12;6(4):e565

Broom GM, Shaw IC, Rucklidge JJ. The ketogenic diet as a potential treatment and prevention strategy for Alzheimer's disease. Nutrition 2019 Apr; 60: 118-121

Burns, Christine M; Chen, Kewei; Kaszniak, Alfred W; Lee, Wendy; Alexander, Gene E; Brandy, Daniel, Fleisher, Adam S; Caselli, Richard J; Reeman, Eric M. Higher serem levels are associated with cerebral hypo metabolism in Alzheimer regions. Neurology 2013 Apr 23; 80(17):1557-1564

Carlson, Anton J; Hoelzel, Frederick. Apparent Prolongation of the Life Span of Rats by Intermittent Fasting: One Figure. The Journal of Nutrition. Volume 31, Issue 3. Marh 1946. page 363-375

Castellano, Christian-Alexandre; Baillargeon, Jean-Patrice; Nugent, Scott; Tremblay, Sebastian; Fortier, Melanie; Imbreault, Helene; Duval Julie; Cunnane, Stephen C. Regional Brain Glucose Hypometabolism in Young Women with Polycystic Ovary Syndrome: Possible Link to Mild Insulin Resistance PLoS One 2015, 10(12) Published online 2015 Dec 9 doi:10.1371/ journal.pope.0144116

Castellaro AM, Tonda A, Cejas HH, et al. Oxalate induces breast cancer. BMC Cancer 2015;15: 761

Chai W, Liebman M. Oxalate content of legumes, nuts and grain-based flours. J Food Compos Anal 2005; 18(7): 723-729

Chen (a) LC, Yang AC, Su TP, Bai YM, Li CT, Chang WH, Chen TJ, Tsai SJ, Chen MH. Symptomatic menopausal transition and subsequent bipolar disorder among midlife women with major depression; a nationwide longitudinal study. <u>Arch Womens Ment Health</u> 2017 Jun;20(3): 463-468

Chen (b)CL, Chou KJ, Wang JS, Yeh JH, Fang HC, Chung HM. Neurotoxic effects of carambola in rats; the role of oxalate. <u>J Formos Med Assoc Taiwan Yi Zhi</u> 2002;101(5):337-341

Cho CE, Tasuwan S, Malysheva OV, Bender E, Tulchinsky NE, Yan J, Sutter JL, Caudill MA. Trimethylamine-N-oxide (TMAO) response to animal source foods varies among healthy men and is influenced by their gut microbiota composition: A randomized controlled trial. <u>Mol Nutr Food Res</u> 20107 Jan;61(1)

Chowdhury R, Warnakula S, Kunutsor S, Crowe F, Ward HA, Johnson L, Franco OH, Butterworth AS, Forouh NG, Thompson SG, Khaw Kt, Mozaffarian D, Danesh J, DiAngelantonio E. Association of dietary, circulating and supplement fatty acids with coronary risk: a systematic review and meta-analysis. <u>Ann Intern Med</u> Mar 18; 160(6):398-406

Christison R, Coindet C. An experimental inquiry on poisoning by oxalic acid. <u>Edinb Med Surg J Exhib Concise View Latest Most Important Discov Med Surg Pharm</u> 1823

Clemens, Zsofia; Daboczi Andrea; Toth, Csaba.   The paleolithic ketogenic diet may ensure adequate serum magnesium levels. Journal of Evolution and Health Vol 2a: Iss 2, Article 6

Cohn, Jay N; Kowey, Peter R; Whelton, Paul K. et al.   Arch Intern Med 2000;160(16) 2429-2436

Coral A, Holsbeeck M, Van Hegg C.   Case report 599: Secondary oxalosis complicating chronic renal failure (oxalate gout).   Skeletal Radiol 1990;19(2): 147-149

Costello, Rebecca B; Elin Ronald J; Rosanoff, Andrea; Wallace, Taylor C, Guerrero-Romero, Fernando; Hruby, Adela; Lutsey, Pamela L; Nielsen Forest H; Rodriguez-Moran, Martha; Song, Yiqing. Perspective: The Case for an Evidence-Based Reference Interval for Serum Magnesium: The Time Has Come. Advances in Nutrition Vol 7 Issue 6, November 2016, Pages 977-993

Craft, Suzanne.   The Role of Metabolic Disorders in Alzheimer's Disease and Vascular Dementia: Two Roads Converged?   Arch Neurol 2009 Mar;77(3); 300-305

Cunnane(a), Stephen C; Coureheane-Loyer, Alexandre; Vanderbeighe, Camille; St Pierre, Valerie; Fortier, Melanie; Hennebelle, Marie; Crolean, Etienne; Bocti Christian; Fulop, James, Castellao, Christian-Alexandre.   Can Ketones Help Rescue Brain Fuel Supply in Later Life? Implications for Cognitive Health During

Aging and the Treatment of Alzheimer's Disease.   Front Mol Neurosci 2016; 9:53

Cunnane(b) SC, Courahesne-Loyer, A; St. Pierre, V; Vanderberghe C; Pierotte T; Fortier M; Croteau E, Castellano CA.   Can ketones compensate for deteriorating brain glucose uptake during aging? Implications for the risk and treatment of Alzheimer's disease. Ann NY Acad Sci 2016 Mar; 1367(1): 12-20

Cunnane(c) SC, Couchesne-Layer A, St-Pierre V, Vanderberghe C, Pierotti T, Fortier M, Croteau E, Castellano CA.   Can ketones compensate for deteriorating brain glucose uptake during aging? Implications for the risk and treatment of Alzheimer's disease. Ann NY Aca Sci 2016 Mar; 1367 (1): 12-20

Cunnane(d) SC, Crawford MA. Energetic and nutritional constraints on infant brain development: implications for brain expansion during human evolution. J Hum Evol 2014 Dec 77:88-98

D'Agostino DP, Pilla R, Held HE, Landon CS, Puchowecz M, Brunengruber H, Ari C, Arnold P, Dean JB. Therapeutic ketosis with ketone ester delays central nervous system oxygen toxicity seizures in rats. Am J Physiol Regul Integr Comp Physiol 20213 May 15;304(10): R829-36

Dashti HM, Mathew TC, Hussein T, Asfar SK, Behbaham A, Khoursheed MA, Al-Saver HM, Bo-Abbas YY, Al-Zaid NS   Long term effects of a ketogenic diet in obese patients. Exp Clin Cardiol 2004 Fall 9(3) 200-205 deAzevedo, Fernanda Reis; Ikeoka, Dimas; Caramelli, Bruno. Effects of intermittent fast on metabolism in men. <u>Revista de Associacao Medica Brasileira</u> Vol 59, Issue 2, March-April 2013, Pages 167-173

DeHaven J, Sherwin R, Hendler R, Felig P. Nitrogen and sodium balance and sympathetic-nervous system activity in obese subjects treated with a low-calorie protein or mixed diet. <u>N Engl J Med</u> 1980 Feb 28; 203(9): 477-82

Descamps O, Riondel J, Ducros V, Roussel AM. Mitochondrial production of reactive oxygen species and incidence of age-related associated lymphoma in OF1 mice: effect of alternate-day fasting. <u>Mech Ageing Dev</u> 2005 Nov; 126(11): 1185-91

deSouza RJ, Mente A, Maroleanu A, Coyma AI, Ha V, Kishibe T, Uleryk E, Budylowski P, Schunemann H, Beyene J, Anand SS. Intake of saturated and trans unsaturated fatty acids and risk of all cause mortality, cardiovascular disease, and type 2 disease: systematic review and meta-analysis of observational studies. <u>BMJ</u> 2015 Aug 11; 351: h3978

DiLorenzo C, Coppola G, Sirianni G, Pierelli F. Short term improvement of migraine headaches during ketogenic diet: a prospective observational study in a dietician clinical setting <u>J Headache Pain</u> 2018; 14(Suppl1): p219

Ede, Georgia. "The Antioxidant Myth" Dec 20, 2017 https://www.psychologytoday.com/us/blog/diagnosis-diet/201/12/the-antioxidant-myth

Eferink JG. The mechanism of calcium oxalate crystal-induced haemolysis of human erythrocytes. Br J Exp Pathol 1987;68(4): 551-557

Ermer T, Eckardt KU, Aronson PS, Knauf F. Oxalate, inflammasome, and progression of kidney disease. Curr Opin Nephrol Hypertens 2016;25(4):363-71

Erol G, Winham SJ, McElroy SL, Frye MA, Prieto ML, Cuellar-Barboza AB, Fuentes M, Geske J, Mori N, Biemacka JM, Bobo WV. Sex differences in the risk of rapid cycling and other indicators of adverse illness course in patients with bipolar I and II disorder. Bipolar Disord 2015 Sep; 17(6): 670-6

Falsetti L, Pasinetti E, Massani MD, Gasialdi A. Weight loss and menstrual cycle: clinical and endocrinological evaluation. Gynecol Endocrinol 1992 Mar; 6(1): 49-56

Faris MA, Kacimi S, Al-Kurd RA; Fararjeh MA, Bustanji YK, Muhammad MK, Salem ML. Intermittent fasting during Ramadan attenuates proinflammatory cytokines and immune cells in healthy subjects. Nutr Res 2012 Dec;32(12)947-55

Fasano(a) A Leaky gut and autoimmune diseases. Clin Rev Allergy Immunol 2012 Feb; 42(1):71-8

Fasano(b) A.   Zonulin and its regulation of intestinal barrier function: the biological door to inflammation, autoimmunity, and cancer. <u>Physical Rev</u> 2011 Jan;91(1): 151-75

Fielder AR, Garner A, Chambers TL. Ophthalmic manifestations of primary oxalosis. <u>Br J Ophthalmol</u> 1980;64(10): 782-788

Fishbein GA, Micheletti RG, Currier JS, Singer E, Fishbein MC. Atherosclerotic Oxalosis in Coronary Arteries. <u>Cardiovasc Pathol Off J Soc Cardiovasc Pathol</u> 1008;17(2):117-123

Fontana, Luigi; Klein, Samuel; Hotlvszy John O; Premachandra, Bhartur N. Effect of Long-term Calorie Restriction with Adequate Protein and Micronutrients on Thyroid Hormones. <u>The Journal of Clinical Endocrinology and Metabolism</u> Vol 91, Issues 8, 1 August 2006, Pages 3232-3235

Freeman MP, Smith KW, Freeman SA, McElroy SL, Kmelz GF, Wright R, Keck PE Jr. The Impact of Reproductive Events on the Course of Bipolar Disorder in Women. <u>J Clin Psychiatry</u> 2002; 63(4) 284-287

Glew RH, Sun Y, Horowitz BL, et al. Nephropathy in dietary hyperoxaluria: A potentially preventable acute or chronic kidney disease. <u>World J Nephrol</u> 2014;3(4):122-142

Goday A, Belido D, Sajoux I, Crujeira AB, Burguera B, Garcia-Luna PP, Oleaga A A, Moreno B, Casanueva FF. Short-term safety, tolerability and efficacy of a very low-calorie ketogenic diet interventional weight loss program versus hypo calorie diet in patients with type 2 diabetes mellitus. <u>Nutr Diabetes</u> 2016 Sep 19;6(9) e230

Goodrick CL, Ingram DK, Reynolds MA, Freeman JR, Cider NL. Effects of Intermittent Feeding Upon Growth and Life Span in Rats. Gerontology 1982; 28: 233-241

Gupta, Ravi; Pathak, Rahid; Bhatia, Manjeet Singh; Banerjee, Basu Del. Comparison of oxidative stress among migraineurs, tension-type headache subjects, and a control group. <u>Ann Indian Acad Neurol</u> 2009 Jul-Sep; 12(3): 167-172

Halton TL, Willett WC, Liu S, Manson JE, Albert CM, Rexrode K, Hu FB. Low-carbohydrate-diet score and the risk of coronary heart disease in women. <u>N Engl J Med</u> 2006 Nov 9;355(19): 1991-2002

Hashim, Sami; Vanitallie, Theodor B. Ketone body therapy: from the ketogenic diet to the oral administration of ketone ester. <u>The Journal of Lipid Research</u> 2014 Sep;55: 1818-1826

Hason-Olive MM, Lauritzen KH, Rasmussen LJ, Storm-Mathisen J, Bergersen LH. A Ketogenic Diet Improves Mitochondrial Biogenesis and Bioenergetics via the PGC1a-SIRT3-UCP2 Axis. <u>Neurochem Res</u> 2019 Jan; 44 (1): 22-37

Hassan MQ, Hadi RA, Al-Rawi ZS, Padron VA, Stohs SS. The glutathione defense system in the pathogenesis of rheumatoid arthritis. J Appl Toxicol 2001 Jan-Feb;21(1): 69-73

Hasselbalch SG, Knudsen GM, Jacobsen J, Hageman LP, Holm S, Paulson OB. Blood brain barrier permeability of glucose and ketone bodies during short-term starvation in humans. Am J Physiol 1995 Jun 268;(6PT1): E116106

Heaney RP, Weaver CM. Oxalate: effect on calcium absorbability. Am J Clin Nutr 1989;50(4): 830-832

Hedemark A, Bang G, Gammeltvedt AT, Anda S. Dental and jaw changes in primary hyperoxaluria. J Oral Pathol Med Off Publ Int Assoc Oral Pathol Am Acad Oral Pathol 1989; 18(10): 586-589

Heianza Y, Ma W, Manson JE, Rexrode KM, Qi L. Gut Microbiota Metabollites and Risk of Major Adverse Cardiovascular Disease Events and Death: A Systematic Review and Meta-Analysis of Prospective Studies. J Am Heart Assoc 2017; Jun 29 6(7)

Henderson ST, Vogel JL, Barr LJ, Garin F, Jones JJ, Constantini LC. Study of the ketogenic agent AC1202 in mild to moderate Alzheimer's disease: a randomized, double blind, placebo-controlled multicenter trial. Nutr Metab (Lond) 2009; 6:31

Ho, Kok-Sun; Tan, Charmane You Mei; David, Makd Ashik Mohd; Seow-Cheon, Francis. Stopping or reducing dietary fiber intake reduces constipation and its associated symptoms. World J Gastroenterol 2012 Sep 7; 18(33):4593-4596

Hollis F, Mitchell ES Canto C, Wong D, Sandi C. Medium chain triglyceride diet reduces anxiety-lie behaviors and enhances social competitiveness in rats. Neuropharmacology 2018 Aug; 138:245-256

Holmes RP, Ambrosius WT, Assimos DG. Dietary oxalate loads and renal oxalate handling. J Urol 2005;174(3):943-947 discussion 947

Howard BV, Van Horn L, Hsia J, Manson JE, Stefanick ML, et al. Low-fat dietary pattern and risk of cardiovascular disease: the Women's Health Initiative Randomized Controlled Dietary Modification Trial. JAMA 2006 Feb 8;295(6): 655-66

Huang, Chou-Long; Kuo, Elizabeth. Mechanism of Hypokalemia in Magnesium Deficiency. JASN October 2007;18(10) 2649-2653

Ishibashi K, Onishi A, Fujiwara Y, Isiwata K, Ishil K. Relationship between Alzheimer's disease-like pattern of 18-F-FDG and fasting plasma glucose levels in cognitively normal volunteers. J Nucl Med 2015 Feb;56(2): 229-33

Isomaa B, Almgren P, Tuomi T, Forsen B, Lahti K, Nissen M, Taskinen MR, Groop L. Cardiovascular morbidity and mortality associated with the metabolic syndrome. Diabetes Care 2001 Apr; 24(4): 683-9

Jahnen-Dechent, Wilhelm; Kettele, Markus.   Magnesium basics. Clin Kidney J 2012 Feb 5 (Suppl 1): i3-i14

Jakobsen MU, Dethiefsen C, Joensen AM, Stegger J, Tionneland A, Schmidt EB, Overvad K.   Intake of carbohydrates compared with intake of saturated fatty acids and risk of myocardial infarction: importance of the glycemic index. Am J Clin Nutr 2010 Jun;91(6): 1764-8

Janssen, Imke; Powell, Lynda H; Crawford, Sybil; Lasley, Bill, Sutton-Tyrrell, Kim.   Menopause and the Metabolic Syndrome. Arch Intern Med 2008 Jul 28;168(4):1568-1575

Jarrett SG, Milder JB, Liang LP.Patel M.   The ketogenic diet increase mitochondrial glutathione levels. J Neurochem 2008 Aug; 106(3): 1044-51

Johnson(a) JB, Summer W, Cutler RG, Martin B, Hyun DH, Dixit VD, Pearson M, Nassar M, Telljohann R, Maudsley S, Carlson O, John S, Laub DR, Mallson MP.   Alternate day calorie restriction improves clinical findings and reduces markers of oxidative stress and inflammation in overweight adults with moderate asthma. Free Radic Biol Med 2007 Mar 1; 42(5):665-74

Johnson(b) J, Short A, Hutchison A, Parrott N, Roberts I.   Small intestinal infarction: a fatal complication of systemic oxalosis. J Clin Pathol 2000;53(9): 720-721

Kamada(a) N, Roger G. The Innate Immune System: A Trigger for Many Chronic Inflammatory Intestinal Diseases.Inflamm Intest Dis 2016;1:70-77

Kamada(b) Nobuhiko; Seo, Sang-Uk; Chen, Grace Y; Nunez, Gabriel. Role of the gut microbiota in immunity and inflammatory disease. Nat Rev Immunol 2013 May; 13(5) 321-335

Katoh R, Suzuki K, Hemmi A, Kawaoi A. Nature and significance of calcium oxalate crystals in normal human thyroid gland. A clinicopathological and immunohistochemical study. Virchows Arch A Pathol Anat Histopathol 1993;422(4):122-142

Kaysen GA, et al. Lipid levels are inversely associated with infectious and all-cause mortality: international MONDO study results. J Lipid Res 2018

Khan SR. Reactive oxygen species, inflammation and calcium oxalate nephrolithiasis. Transl Aandrol Urol 2014;3(3):256-276

Kim DY, Hao J, Liu R, Turner G, Shi FD, Rho JM. Inflammation-mediated memory dysfunction and effects of a ketogenic diet in a murine model of multiple sclerosis. PLoS One 2012; 7(5): e35476

Kim I, Lemasters JJ. Mitochondrial degradation by autophagy (mitophagy) in GFP-LC3 transgenic hepatocytes during nutrient deprivation. Am J Physiol Cell Physiol 2011 Feb;200(2) c308-17

Klement RJ, Pazienza V. Impact of Different Types of Diet on Gut Microbiota Profiles and Cancer Prevention and Treatment. Medicena (Kaunas) 2019 Mar 29: 55 (4)

Konig J, Wells J, Cani PD, Garcia-Rodenas CL, MacDonald T, Mercenier A, Whyte J, Troost F, Brummer RJ. Human Intestinal Barrier Function in Health and Disease. Clin Transl Gastroenterol 2016 Oct 20;7(10):e196

Kopp, Wolfgang. Nutrition, evolution and thyroid hormone levels— a link to iodine deficiency disorders? Medical Hypothesis. 2004 June 04; Vol 62, Iss 6: 871-875

Kovacs Z, D'Agostino DP, Diamond D, Kindy MS, Rogers C, An, C. Therapeutic Potential of Exogenous Ketone Supplement Induced Ketosis in the Treatment of Psychiatric Disorders: Review of Current Literature. Front Psychiatry 2019; 10:363

Landfold Bjarno; Valeur, Jorgen; Berstad, Arnold; Raa, Jan. Microbial trimethylamine-N-oxide as a disease marker: something fishy? Microb Ecol Health Dis 2017; 28(1): 1327309

Lapointe HJ, Listrom R. Oral manifestations of oxalosis secondary to ileojejunal intestinal by pass. Oral Surg Oral Med Oral Pathol 1988;65(1):76-80

Lee C, Raffaghello L, Brandhorst S, Salfdie FM, Branchi G, Martin-Montalvo A, Pistoia V, Wei M, Hwang S, Merino A, Emionele L, deCabo R, Longo VD. Fasting cycles retard growth of tumors and sensitize a range of cancer cell types to chemotherapy. Sci Transl Med 2012 Mar 7; 4(124):124ra27

Lewis LD, Smith BW, Mamourian AC. Delayed sequelae after acute overdoses or poisonings: cranial neuropathy related to ethylene glycol ingestion. Clin Pharmacol Ther 1997;61(6): 692-699

Liang Y, Vetrano DL, Qiu C. Serum total cholesterol and risk of cardiovascular and non-cardiovascular mortality in old age: a population-based study. BMC Geriatr 2017 Dec 28;17(1): 294

Longo, Valter D; Mallson, Mark. Fasting: Molecular Mechanisms and Clinical Applications. Cell Metab 2014 Jan 16

Maalouf(a), Marwan; Rho, Jong M; Mattson, Mar P. The neuroprotective properties of calorie restriction, the ketogenic diet, and ketone bodies. Brain Res Rev Vol 59 Iss 2, Mar 09: 293-315

Maalouf(b), Marwan; Sullivan, Patrick G; Davis, Laurie; Kim, DoYoung; Rho, Johg M. Ketones Inhibit Mitochondrial Production of Reactive Oxygen Species Production Following Glutamate Excitotoxicity by Increasing NADH Oxidation. Neuroscience 20007 Mar 2; 145 (1): 256-264

Magnesium. Dietary Reference Intakes for Calcium, Phosphorus, Magnesium, Vitamin D and Fluoride (1997) Chapter: 6 Magnesium. The National Academies Press NAP.edu/10766

Maldonado I, Prasad V, Reginato AJ. Oxalate crystal deposition disease. <u>Curr Rheumatol Rep</u> 2002;4(3):257-264

Malik S, Wong W, Franklin SS, Kamath TV, L'Italien GL, Pio JR, Williams GR. Impact of the metabolic syndrome on mortality from coronary heart disease, cardiovascular disease and all causes in United States adults. <u>Circulation</u> 2004 Sept 7; 110(10):1245-50

Mansell, PI, Fellows, IW, MacDonald IA. Enhanced thermogenic response to epinephrine after 48-h starvation in humans. <u>Am J Physiol</u> 1990 Jan; 258(1PT2):R87-93

Marconi V, Mofid MZ, McCall C, Eckman I, Nousari HC. Primary hyperoxaluria: report of a patient with livedo reticularis and digital infarcts. <u>J Am Acad Dermatol</u> 1001;46(2 Suppl Case Reports):S16-18

Martensson, Johannes; Han, Jihong; Griffith, Gwen W; Meister, Alton. Glutathione ester delays the onset of scurvy in ascorbate-deficient guinea pigs. <u>Proc Nat Acad Sci USA</u> Jan 1993; Vol 90: 317-321,

Mathieson, Ruth A; Walbert, Janet L; Gwazdauskas, Francis C; Hinkle, Dennis E; Gregg, John M.   The effect of varying carbohydrate content of a very-low-calorie-diet on resting metabolic rate and thyroid hormones. <u>Metabolism</u> Vol 35; Iss 5, May 1986: 394-398

Matsuzaki T, Sasaki K, Tanizaki Y, Hata J, Fujimi K, Matsui Y, Sokita A, Suzuki SO, Kanba S, Koyohara Y, Iwaki T. Insulin resistance is associated with the pathology of Alzheimer disease: the Hisayama study. <u>Neurolgy</u> 2010; Aug 331;75(9):764-70

Mattson MP. Energy intake, meal frequency, and health: a neurobiological perspective. <u>Annu Rev Nutr</u> 2005; 25:237-60

Mavropoulos, John C; Yancy, William S; Hapburn, Juanity; Westman, Eric C. The effects of a low-carbohydrate, ketogenic diet in the polycystic ovary syndrome: a pilot study. <u>Nutr Metab (Long)</u> 2004;2:35

McGrice, Melance; Porter, Judi. The Effects of Low Carbohydrate Diets on Fertility Hormones and Outcomes in Overweight and Obese Women: A Systematic Review. <u>Nutrients</u> 2017 Feb 27 (9)3

Mehendale HM. Toxicodynamics of low level toxicant interactions of biological significance: inhibition of tissue repair. <u>Toxicology</u> 1995;105(2-3):251-266

Mehrabanii H, Hamayeli; Salehpaur S; Amiri Z; Farahani, S Jalali; Meyer, BJ; Tahbaz, F. Beneficial effects of a high protein, low-glycemic-load hypo caloric diet in overweight and obese women with polycystic ovary syndrome: a randomized controlled intervention study. <u>J Am Coll Nutr</u> 31 (2):117-125

Mente A, deKoning L, Shannon HS, Anand SS. A systematic review of the evidence supporting a causal link between dietary factors and coronary heart disease. <u>Arch Intern Med 2009 Apr 13;169(7): 659-69</u>

Metzner, Helmut; Bourne, Geoffrey. Vitamin C in the Animal Cell (Die Ascorbinsaure in de Pflanzenzelle). Pub: Springer

Mielke(a) MM, Zandi PP, Shao H, Waem M, et al. The 32-year relationship between cholesterol and dementia from midlife to late life. <u>Neurology</u> 2010 Nov 23; 75(21): 1888-1895

Mielke(b) MM, Zandi PP, Sjogren M, Gustafson D, Ostline S, Steen B, Skoog I. High total cholesterol levels in late life associated with a reduced risk of dementia. <u>Neurology April 20, 2005</u>

Milder, Julie B; Patel, Manisha. Modulation of oxidative stress and mitochondrial function by the ketogenic diet. <u>Epilepsy Res</u> 2012 Jul; 100(3):295-303

Miller, Vincent J; Hyde, Parker N; Dickerson, Ryan; LaFountain, Richard A; Maresh, Carl M; Kraemer, William J; Volek, Jeff. The Ketogenic Diet Alters Endocrine Regulation of Energy Metabolism in Ultra-Endurance Athletes. <u>FASEB Journal</u> 2017 Apr 1; Abstract Nbr 1036.3

Mohorko N, Cernelic-Bizjak M, Poklar-Vatovec T, Grom G, Kenig S, Petelin A, Jenko-Praznikar Z. Weight loss, improved physical performance, cognitive function, eating behavior, and metabolic profile in a 12-week ketogenic diet in obese adults. <u>Nutr Res</u> 2019 Feb; 62:64-77

Moorhead PJ, Cooper DJ, Timperley WR. Progressive peripheral neuropathy in patient with primary hyperoxaluria   Br Med J 1975;2(5966): 312-313

Moskow BS.   Periodontal manifestations of hyperoxaluria and oxalises. J Periodontol 1989;60(5):271-278

Mulay SR, Desai J, Kumar SV, et al.   Cytotoxicity of crystals involves RIPK3-MLKL-mediated necroptosis.   Nat Commun 2016;7:10274

Murphy P, Lekhodii S, Nylen K, Burnham WM. The antidepressant properties of the ketogenic diet.   Biol Psychiatry 2004 Dec 15;56(12):981-83

Nair, Pradeep MK; Khawale, Pranan G. Role of therapeutic fasting in women's health: An overview J Midlife Health 2016 Apr-Jun;7(2): 61-64

Norton, Sally K. Lost Seasonality and Overconsumption of Plants: Risking Oxalate Toxicity. Journal of Evolution and Health Vol 2: Iss 3, Article 4

O'Hearn, L. Amber.   C is for Carnivore   Empirica www.empiri.ca/ 20107102/c-is-for-carnivore.html

Olson, MB, Kelsey SF, Matthews KA, Merz CNB, Eteiba W, McGorray SP, Cornell CE, Vido DA, Uldoon MF. Lipid-Lowering

Medication Use and Aggression Scores in Women: A Report from the NHLBI-Sponsored WISE Study. J Womens Health (Larchmt) 2008 Mar; 17(2) 187-194

Pacchiarohi I, Leon-Caballero J, Murra A, Verdelini N, Furio MA, Pancheri C, Valenti M, Samalin L, Roige ES, Gonzalex-Pinto A, Montes JM, Benabarre A, Crespo JM, de Dios Perinno C, Goikolea JM, Gutieriez-Rojas L, Carvalhoaf, Vieta E. Mood stabilizers and antipsychotics during breastfeeding.   Focus on bipolar disorder. Eur Neuropsychopharmacol 2016 Oct; 26(10):1562-78

Paddock C. High cholesterol diagnosis tied to lower breast cancer risk.   Medical News Today 30 August 2017 https:// www.medicalnewstoday.com/articles/319199.php

Panis V, Tosios KI, Gagari E, Griffin TJ, Damoulis PD.   Severe periodontitis in a patient with hyperoxaluria and oxalosis: a case report and review of the literature.   J Periodontol 2010;81(10): 1497-1504

Paoli A, Rubini A, Volek JA, Grimaldi KA. Beyond weight loss: a review of the therapeutic uses of very-low-carbohydrate (ketogenic) diets. Eur J Clin Nutr 2013 Aug;67(8):789-796

Pasquali R, Parenti M, Mattioli L, Capelli M, Cavazzeni G, Baraldi G, DeBenedettis G, Biso P, Melchionda N.   Effect of dietary carbohydrates during hypocaloric treatment of obesity on peripheral thyroid hormone metabolism.   J Endocrinol Invest 1982 Jan-Feb; 5(1):47-52

Peery AF, Sandler RS.   Diverticular disease: reconsidering conventional wisdom.   Clin Gastroenterol Hepatol 2013 Dec; 11(12):1532-7

Perich TA, Roberts G, Frankland A, Sinbandhit C, Meade T, Austin MP, Mitchell PB.   Clinical characteristics of women with cycle-associated bipolar disorder symptoms.   Aust NZJ Psychiatry 2017 Feb; 51(2):161-167

Perugi G, Medda P, Toni C, Mariani MG, Socci C, Mauri M.   The Role of Electroconvoulsive Therapy (ECT) in Bipolar Disorder: Effectiveness in 522 Patients with Bipolar Depression, Mixed-state, Mania and Catatonic Features.   Curr Neurpharmacol 2017 Apr; 15(3) 359-371

Phelps Jr, Siemers SV, El-Mallakh RS.   The ketogenic diet for type II bipolar disorder.   Neuropharmacol 2013;19(5) 423-6

Phinney, Stephen D.   Ketogenic diets and physical performance. Vol 1, Article nbr 2 (2004) Nutr Metab (Lond) 2004; Aug 17 1(1):2

Pinto A, Bonucci A, Maggi E, Corsi M, Businaro R. Antioxidant and Anti-inflammatory Activity of Ketogenic Diet: New Perspectives for Neuroprotection in Alzheimer's Disease. Antioxidants (Basel) 2018 Apr 28; 7 (5)

Poff AM, Ward N, Seyfried TN, Arnold P, D'Agostino DP. Non-toxic Metabolic Management of Metastic Cancer in VM Mice: Novel

Combination of Ketogenic Diet, Ketone Supplementation and Hyperbaric Oxygen Therapy. PLoS One 2015 Jun 10; 10(6):e0127407

Potassium. Dietary Reference Intakes for Water, Potassium, Sodium, Chloride and Sulphate (2005) Chapter:5 Potassium. The National Academies Press NAP.edu/10766

Price KD, Price CS, Reynolds RD. Hypoglycemia-induced ascorbic acid deficiency promotes endothelial dysfunction and the development of atherosclerosis. Atherosclerosis 2001 Sep;158(1): 1012

Radi MJ. Calcium oxalate crystals in breast biopsies. An overlooked form of micro calcification associated with benign breast disease. Arch Pathol Lab Med 1989;113(12): 1367-1369

Rahman SS, Kadakia S, Balsam L, Rubinstein S. Autonomic dysfunction as a delayed sequelae of acute ethylene glycol ingestion: a case report and review of the literature. J Med Toxicol Off J Am Coll Med Toxicol 2012:8(2):124-129

Ravnskov(a) U, deLorgeril M, Diamond DM, Hama R, Hamazaki T, Hammarskjold B. LDL-C does not cause cardiovascular disease: a comprehensive review of the current literature. J Expert Review of Clinical Pharmacology Vol 11, 2018: Issue 10

Ravnskov(b) U, et al.   High cholesterol may protect against infections and atherosclerosis. QJMVol 96, Iss 12; Dec 2003: 927-933

Rebello CJ, Keller JN, Liu AG, Johnson WD, Greenway FL.   Pilot feasibility and safety study examining the effect of medium chain triglyceride supplementation in subjects in mild cognitive impairment. A randomized controlled trial. BBA Clin 2015 Jan 16; 3:123-5

Recober, Ana; Peterlin, B Lee.   Migraine and obesity: moving beyond BMZ. Future Neurol 2014 Jan 1:9(1)1 37-40

Regenold WR, Phatak P, Makley MT, Stone RD, Kling MA. Cerebrospinal fluid evidence of increased extra-mitochondrial glucose metabolism implicates mitochondrial dysfunction in multiple sclerosis disease progression. J Neurol Sci 2008 Dec 15; 275(1-2): 106-12

Reginato AJ.   Calcium Oxalate and Other Crystals or Particles Associated with Arthritis. In: Koopman WJ, editor. Arthritis and Allied Conditions.   Philadelphia, PA [etc]: Lippincott Williams & Wilkins; 2001

Rhyu, Hgun-seung; Cho, Su-Youn; Roh, Hee-Tae.   The effects of ketogenic diet on oxidative stress and anti oxidative capacity markers of Taekwondo athletes. J Exerc Rehabil 2014 Dec;10(6): 362-366

Richelson B, Pedersen SB.   Associations below different anthropometric measurements of fatness and metabolic risk parameters in non-obese, healthy, middle-aged men. <u>Int J Obes Relat Metab Disord</u> 1995 Mar; 19(3):169-174

Robb JC, Young LT, Cooke RG, Joffe RT. Gender differences in patients with bipolar disorder influence outcome in the medical outcomes survey (SF-20) sub scale scores. <u>J Affect Disord</u> 1998 Jun; 49(3):189-93

Rocha NS, Barbison LF, deOliviera ML, deCamargo JL. Effects of fasting and intermittent fasting on rat hepatocarcinogenesis induced by diethylnitrosamine.   <u>Teratog Carcinog Mutagen</u> 2002; 22(2): 129-38

Rogawski, Michael A.   Migraine and Epilepsy—Shared Mechanisms within the Family of Episodic Disorders. Noebals JL, Avol M, Rogawski MA, et al editors. Jasper's Basic Mechanisms of the Epilepsies. 4th edition.   Bethesda (MD): National Center for Biotechnology Information (US); 2012

Ronnemaa E, Zethelius B, Sundelof J, Degerman-Gunnarsson M, Berne C, Lannfelt L, Kelander L.   Impaired insulin secretion increases the risk of Alzheimer disease. Neurology 2008 Sept 30; 71 (14): 1065-71

Rose DP, Boyar AP, Cohen C, Strong E. Effect of a low-fat diet on hormone levels in women with cystic breast disease. I. Serum steroids and gonadotropins. <u>J Natl Cancer Inst</u> 1987 Apr; 78(4): 623-6

Rubinstein MC, Martinelli PT, Bayer-Garner IB, Klebuc MJ, Curry JL, Hsu S. Persistent cutaneous manifestations of hyperoxaluria after combined hepatorenal transplantation. <u>Dermatol Online J</u> 2004; 10(1)

Rude, Robert K. Magnesium Deficiency: A Cause of Heterogenous Disease in Humans. <u>J Bone Min Res</u> 1998 Vol 13 Nbr 4

Sadiya A, Ahmed S, Siddieg HH, Babas IJ, Carisson M. Effect of Ramadan fasting on metabolic markers, body composition, and dietary intake in Emirates of Ajman (UAE) with metabolic syndrome. <u>Diabetes Metab Syndr Obes</u> 2011; 4: 409-416

Salyer WR, Hutchins GM. Cardiac lesions in secondary oxalosis. <u>Arch Intern Med</u> 1974; 134(2): 250-252

Samarneh MM, Shtaynberg N, Goldman M, Epstein E, Kleiner M, El-Sayegh S. Severe oxalosis with systemic manifestations. <u>J Clin Med Res</u> 2012; 4(1):56-60

Sansone, Randy A. Cholesterol Quandaries: Relationship to Depression and the Suicidal Experience. <u>Psychiatry (Edgmont)</u> 2008 Mar; 5(3): 22-34

Saslow LR, Mason AE, Kim S, Goldman V, Ploutz-Snyder R, Bayandorian H, Daubenmier J, Hecht FM, Moskowitz JT. An Online

Intervention Comparing a Very Low-Carbohydrate Diet in Overweight Individuals with Type 2 Diabetes: A Randomized Controlled Trial. <u>J Med Internet Res</u> 2017 Feb 13; 19(2): e36

Saunders, Ericka FH; Fitzgerald, Kate D; Zhang, Peng; Mcinnis, Melvin G. Clinical Features of Bipolar Disorder Comorbid with Anxiety Disorders Differ Between Men and Women. <u>Depress Anxiety</u> 2012 Aug: 29(8): 739-746

Schrijvers EM, Witteman JC, Sijbrands EJ, Hofman A, Koudstaal PJ, Brateler MM. Insulin metabolism and the risk of Alzheimer disease: the Rotterdam Study. <u>Neurology</u> 2010 Nov 30; 75(22): 19827

Seippel L, Backstrom T. Luteal-phase estradiol relates to symptom severity in patients with premenstrual syndrome. <u>J Clin Endocrinol Metab</u> 1998 Jun; 83(6):1988-92

Sharman MJ, Kraemer WJ, Love DM, Avery NG, Gomez AL, Scheet TP, Volek JS. A ketogenic diet favorably affects serum biomarkers for cardiovascular disease in normal-weight men. <u>J Nutr</u> 2002 Jul; 132 (7):1879-85

Shavit L, Girfoglio D, Vijay V, et al. Vascular calcification and bone mineral density in recurrent kidney stone formers. <u>Clin J Am Soc Nephrol CJASN</u> 2015; 10(2): 278-285

Sherman H, Genzer Y, Cohen R, Chapruk N, Madar Z, Froy O. Timed high-fat diet resets circadian metabolism and prevents obesity. <u>FASEB</u> 2012 Aug 26 (8) 3493-502

Siener R, Honow R, Voss S, Seidler A, Hesse A. Oxalate content of cereals and cereal products. <u>J Agric Food Chem</u> 2006; 54(8): 3008-3011

Siri-Tarino PW, Sun Q, Fuf B, Krauss RM.   Meta-analysis of prospective fat cohort studies evaluation the association of saturated fat with cardiovascular disease. <u>Am J Clin Nutr</u> 2010 Mar 9; 91 (3): 535-46

Sit, Dorothy. Women and Bipolar Disorder Across the Life Span <u>J Am Med Womens Assoc</u> 2004 Spring;59(2): 91-100

Sogawa, Hiroshi; Kubo Chiharu. Influence of short-term repeated fasting on the longevity of female (NZB x NZW) F1 mice. <u>Mechanisms of Aging and Development</u> Vol 115, Issues 102 17 May 2000: 61-71

Spadaro PA, Naug HL DuToit EF, Donner D, Colson NI. A refined high carbohydrate diet is associated with changes in the serotonin pathway and visceral obesity. <u>Genet Res (Camb)</u> 2015 Dec 28: 97 e 23

Spencer J, Hibberd TJ, Travis L, Wiklendt L, Costa M, Hu H, Brookes SJ, Wattchow DA, Dinning PG, Keating DJ, Sorensen J. Identification of a Rhythmic Firing Pattern in the Enteric Nervous

System that Generates Rhythmic Electrical Activity in Smooth Muscle. <u>J of Neuros</u> 13 June 2018 38 (24) 5508-5522

Storoni, Mithu; Plant, Gordon T. The Therapeutic Potential of the Ketogenic Diet in Treating Progressive Multiple Sclerosis. <u>Mult Scle Int</u> 2015, 2015.681289

Strijbis, Karin; Vaz, Frediric M; Distel Ben. Enzymology of the carnitine biosynthesis pathway. <u>IVBMB Life</u> 2018 May 62 (5) 357-62

Stubbs, BJ, Cox PJ, Evans RD, Sarter P, Miller JJ, Faull OK, Magor-Ellott S, Hiyama S Stirling M, Clarke K. On the Metabolism of Exogenous Ketones in Humans. <u>Front Physiol</u> 2017;8:848

Sun, X-Y, Ouyang J-M, Zhu W-Y, Li Y-B, Gan Q-Z. Size-dependent toxicity and interactions of calcium oxalate dihydrate crystals on Vero renal epithelial cells. <u>J Mater Chem B</u> 2015;3(9): 1974-1878

Synmans PJ, Brady K, Keen CE. Calcium oxalate crystal deposition in epitheloid histiocytes of granulomatous lymphadenitis: analysis by light and electron microscopy. <u>Histopathology</u> 1995;27(5): 423-429

Tan, KY, Seow-Choen F. Fiber and colorectal disease: separating fact from fiction <u>World J Gastroenterol</u> 2007 Aug 21; 13(31): 4161-7

Teatero ML, Mazmaman D, Sharma V.   Effects of the menstrual cycle on bipolar disorder. <u>Bipolar Disord</u> 2014 Feb;16(1): 22-36

Toth, Csaba; Daboczi, Andrea; Howard, Mark; Miller, Nicholas; Clemens, Zsofia.   Crohn's disease successfully treated with the paleolithic ketogenic diet.   <u>Int J Case Rep Images</u>   2016:7(10) 570-578

Tsai M-H, Chang, W-N, Lui C-C, et al.   Status epilepticus induced by star fruit intoxication in patients with chronic renal disease. <u>Seizure - Eur J Epilepsy</u> 2004;14(7): 521-525

Varady KA, Bhutani S, Church EC, Klempel MC.   Short term modified alternate-day fasting: a novel dietary strategy for weight loss and cardio protection in obese adults.   <u>Am J Clin Nutr</u> 2009 Nov; 90 (5): 1138-43

Viguera AC, Tondo L, Koukopoulos AE, Reginaldi D, Lepri B, Baldessarini RJ. Episodes of mood disorders in 2,252 pregnancies and postpartum periods.   <u>Am J Psychiatry</u> 2011 Nov;168(11): 1179-85

Volek(a) JS, Sharman MJ, Love DM, Avery NG, Gomez AL, Scheet TP, Kraemer WJ. Body composition and hormonal responses to a carbohydrate-restricted diet. <u>Metabolism</u> 2002 Jul;51(7): 864-70

Volek(b), Jeff S; Kraemer William J, Bush, Jill A; Incledon, Thomas; Boltes, Mark.   Testosterone and cortisol in relationship to dietary nutrients and resistance exercise. <u>www.physiology.org/journal/jappl</u>

Volek(c) JS Sharman MJ, Forsythe CE. Modification of lipoproteins by very low-carbohydrate diets. J Nutr 2005 Jun;135(6): 1339-42

Volek(d) JS, Fernandez ML, Feinman RD, Phinney SD. Dietary carbohydrate restriction induces a unique metabolic state positively affecting atherogenic dyslipidemia fatty acid partitioning and metabolic syndrome. Progress in Lpid Research 47 (2008) 307-318

Weiner RD, Reti IM. Key updates in the clinical application of electroconvulsive therapy. Int Rev Psychiatry 2017 Apr; 29(2): 54-62

Wang(a) Z, Bergeron N, Levison BS, Li XS, Chiu S, Jia X, Koeth RA, Li L, Wu Y, Tang WHW, Krauss RM, Hazen SL. Impact of chronic dietary red meat, white meat, or non meat protein on trimethylamin-N-oxide metabolism and renal excretion in healthy men and women. Eur Heart J 2918 Feb 14;40(7): 583-594

Wang(b) Z, Tangella K, Balla A, Popescu G. Tissue refractive index as marker of disease. Biomed Opt [Internet] 2011 [cited 2015 Jun 16]; 16(11)
http://www.ncbi.nlm.nih.gov/pmc/articles/PMC3223513/

Westerman S, Wenger NK. Women and heart disease the under recognized burden: sex differences, biases, and unmet clinical and research challenges. Clin Sci (Lond) 2016 Apr; 130(8): 551-63

Westman EC, Tondit J, Maguire E, Yancy WS Jr. Implementing a low-carbohydrate, ketogenic diet to manage type 2 diabetes mellitus. <u>Expert Rev Endocrinol Metab</u> 2018 Sep; 13(5): 263-272

Whang, Robert; Ryder, Kenneth W. Frequency of Hypomagnesemia and Hypermagnesemia. <u>JAMA</u> 1990; 263(22): 3063-3064

Wheless, James. History of the Ketogenic Diet. <u>Epilepsia</u> 2008 N0049 Suppl 8: 3-5

Williams TJ, Cervenka MC. The role for ketogenic diets in epilepsy and status epilepticus in adults. <u>Clin Neurophysiol Pract</u> 2017 1;2: 154-160

Yamanashi T, Iwata M, Kamiya N, Tsunetomi K, Kajitani N, Wada N, Iitsuka T, Yumauchi T, Miura A, Pu S, Shirayama Y, Watanabe K, Duman RS, Kaneko K. Beta hydroxybutyrate, an endogic NLRP3 inflammasome inhibitor, attenuates stress-induced behavior and inflammatory responses. <u>Sci Rep</u> 2017 Aug 9;7(1):7677

Youm YH, Nguyen KY, Grant RW, Goldberg EL, Bodogai M, Kim D, D'Agostino, Planavsky N, Lupfer C, Kanneganti TD, Kang S, Horvath TL, Fahmy TM, Crawford PA, Bragyn A, Alnemri E, Dixit VD. The ketone metabolite B-hydroxybutyrate blocks NLRP3 inflammasome-mediated inflammatory disease. <u>Nat Med</u> 2015 Mar;21(3): 263-9

Zarate, Sandra; Stevnsner, Tinna; Gredilla, Ricardo.   Role of Estrogen and Other Six Hormones in Brain Aging Neuroprotection and DNA Repair. <u>Front Aging Neurosci</u> 2017, 9: 430

Zauner C, Schneeweiss B, Krantz A, Madi C, Ratheiser K, Kramer L, Roth E, Schneide B, Lenz K.   Resting energy expenditure in short-term starvation is increased as a result of an increase in serum norepinephrine. <u>Am J Clin Nutr</u> 2000 Jun; 71(6): 1511-5

Zhang H, Fu R, Guo C, Huang Y, Wang H, Wang S, Zhao J, Yang N.   Anti-dsDNA antibodies bind to TLR4 and activates NLRP3 inflammasome in lupus monocytes/macrophages.   <u>J Transi Med</u> 2016; 14: 156

About the Author

Claudia Drake has an undergraduate degree in Government and English, as well as a Master's Degree in Public Administration from Eastern Washington University. As a gift to herself in mid-life, she obtained a Master of Arts in Philosophy and Religion, specifically in Women's Spirituality, from the California Institute of Integral Studies, San Francisco, CA. She resides in a small town in southwestern Washington state.

www.ingramcontent.com/pod-product-compliance
Lightning Source LLC
Chambersburg PA
CBHW031236250726
48655CB00005B/1975